THE COMPLETE GALVESTON DIET FOR BEGINNERS

1200 Days Of Essential Low Carb, Anti-Inflammatory Recipes And The Foolproof

Intermittent Fasting Diet Plan With Full Color Pictures

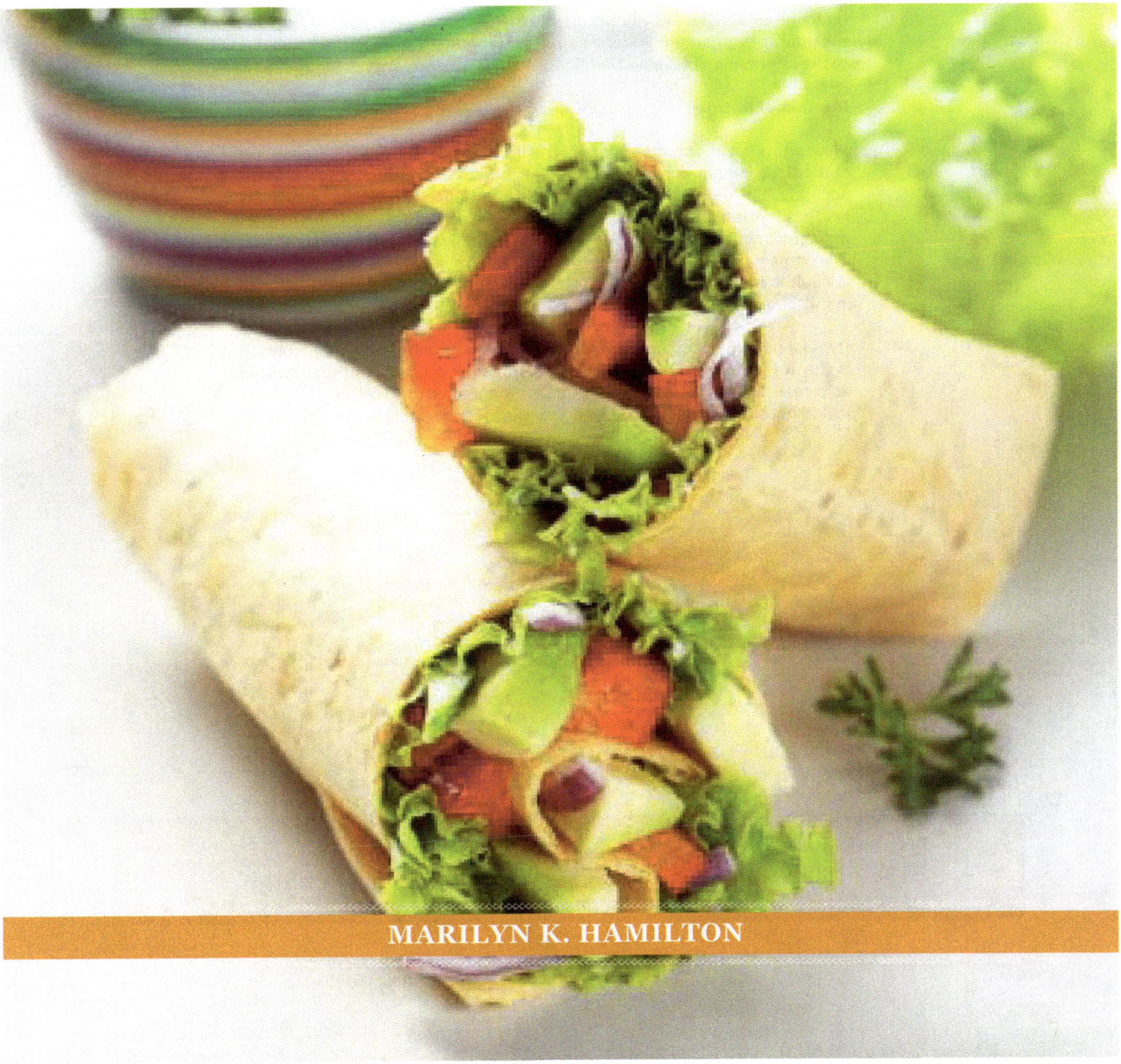

MARILYN K. HAMILTON

EDITOR: LYN

COVER ART: ABR

INTERIOR DESIGN: FAIZAN

FOOD STYLIST: JO

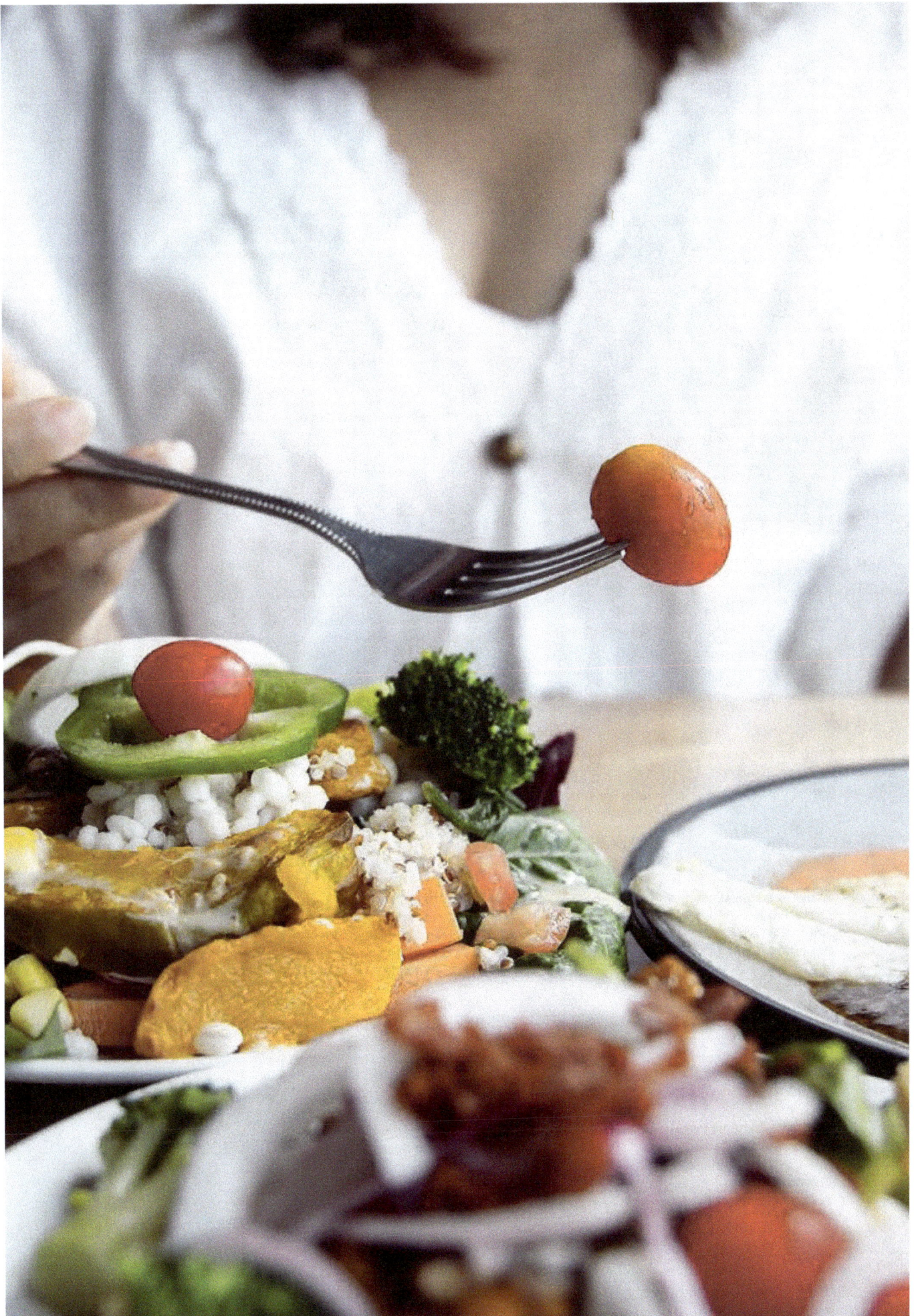

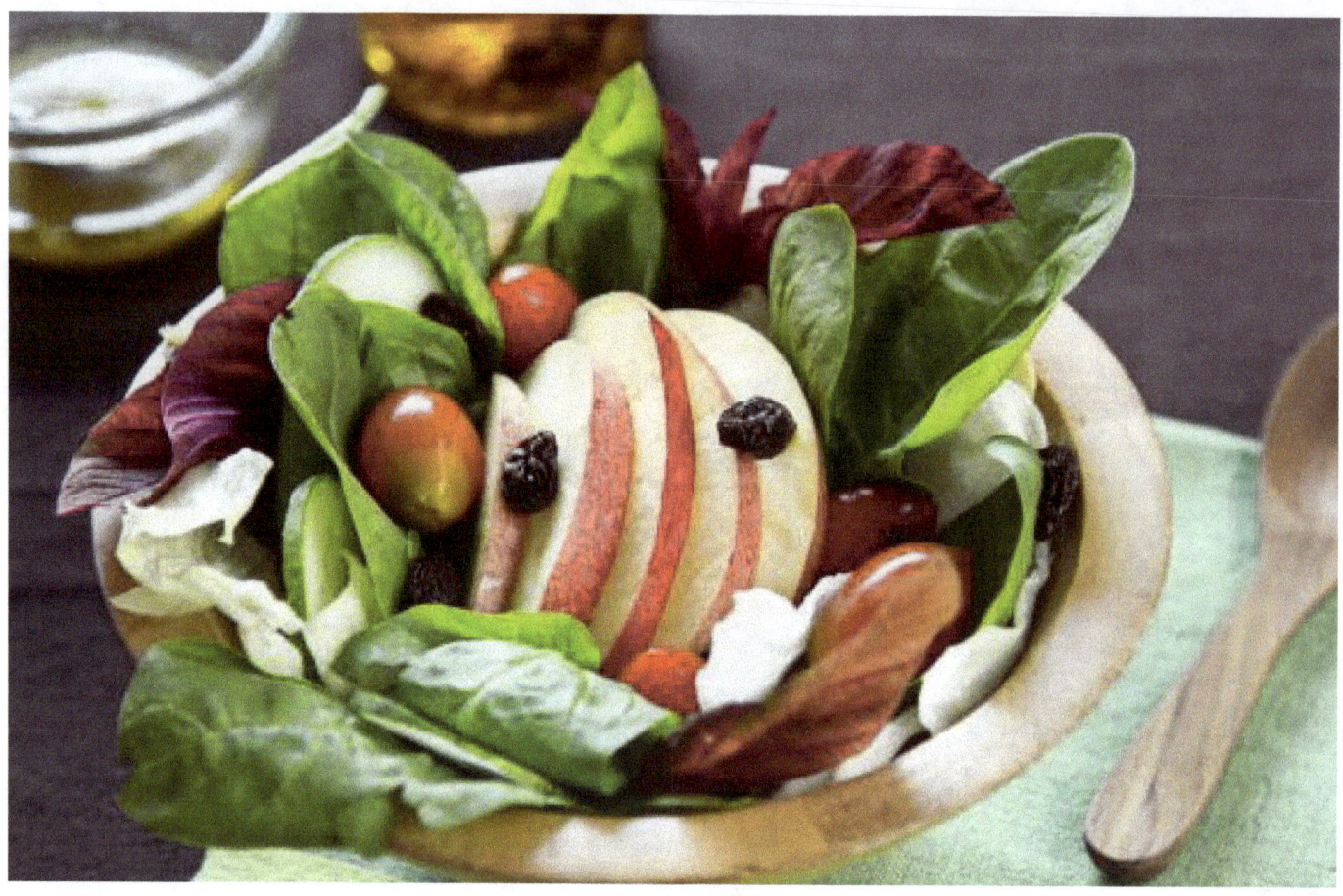

Table of Contents

Introduction

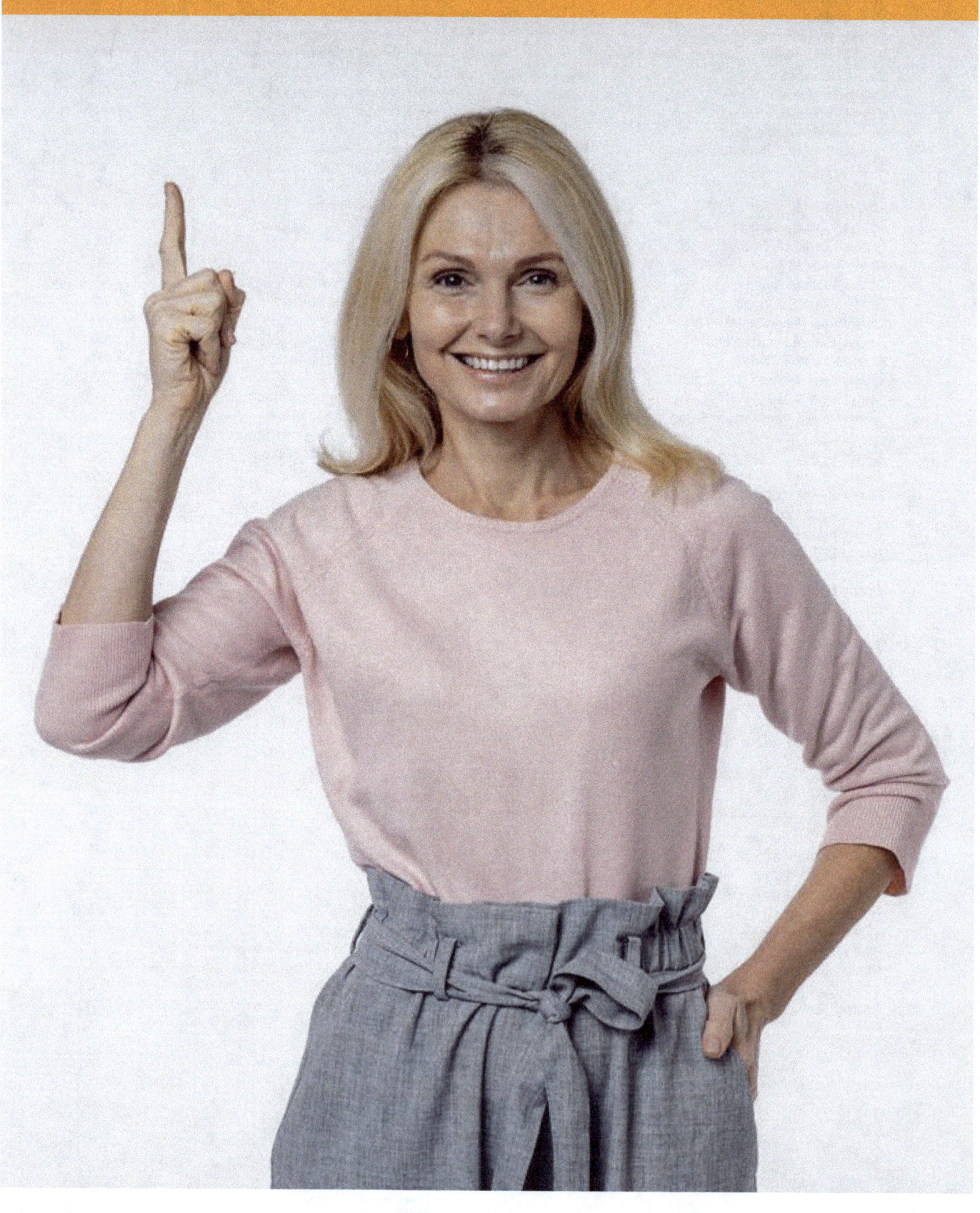

The Galveston diet is a popular eating plan designed specifically for women over 40. It was created by Dr. Mary Claire Haver, a board-certified obstetrician and gynecologist who noticed that many of her patients were struggling with weight loss and hormonal imbalances as they aged.

The Galveston diet emphasizes whole foods, healthy fats, and protein while limiting carbohydrates and processed foods. It also takes into account women's unique hormonal needs, with specific recommendations for supplements and lifestyle changes that can support healthy hormone balance. Many women have reported successful weight loss and improved health on the Galveston diet.

In addition, the Galveston diet has been featured in several media outlets, including television shows and magazines, which has helped to increase its visibility and popularity.

Chapter 1
Your Changing Body, Your Changing Needs

Middle-aged women often face a number of physical changes that can be challenging to manage. Menopause, which typically occurs in a woman's 40s or 50s, is one of the most significant changes that women experience during this time. Menopause marks the end of a woman's reproductive years and is defined by the cessation of menstruation. During this time, women may experience a range of symptoms, including hot flashes, mood swings, vaginal dryness, and weight gain.

One of the primary reasons that women experience these changes is due to changes in their hormone levels. Estrogen levels, in particular, decline during menopause, which can lead to a range of physical and emotional symptoms. Women may also experience changes in their metabolism and muscle mass, which can contribute to weight gain and difficulty maintaining muscle tone.

In addition to menopause, middle-aged women may also face other physical changes related to aging. For example, bone density tends to decline as women age, which can increase the risk of fractures and other injuries. Women may also experience changes in their skin, such as decreased elasticity and wrinkles, as well as changes in their vision and hearing.

Managing these physical changes can be challenging, but there are steps that women can take to support their health and well-being during this time. Eating a healthy diet, engaging in regular exercise, and getting enough sleep are all important for maintaining overall health and managing weight gain. Hormone replacement therapy (HRT) may also be an option for women who are struggling with severe symptoms related to menopause.

Overall, the physical changes that middle-aged women face can be difficult to navigate, but with the right support and care, women can manage their symptoms and maintain their health and well-being. It's important to talk to a healthcare provider about any concerns or symptoms that arise during this time and to seek treatment as needed.

Perimenopause

Perimenopause is the period of time leading up to menopause, during which a woman's hormone levels begin to fluctuate and her body prepares for the end of her reproductive years. Perimenopause can last for several years, and is typically characterized by irregular menstrual cycles, as well as symptoms such as hot flashes, mood swings, and vaginal dryness. During perimenopause, estrogen levels begin to decline, which can lead to changes in a woman's body and overall health.

While perimenopause is a natural and normal process that all women go through, it can be challenging to manage for some women. The symptoms of perimenopause can be disruptive and uncomfortable, and can affect a woman's quality of life. However, there are several strategies that women can use to manage their symptoms during this time. For example, making dietary changes such as reducing caffeine and alcohol intake, exercising regularly, and getting enough sleep can all help to manage hot flashes and mood swings.

SYMPTOMS IN PERIMENOPAUSE

Irregular menstrual cycles: One of the most notable symptoms of perimenopause is changes in menstrual cycles. Women may experience shorter or longer cycles, heavier or lighter bleeding, or skipped periods.

Hot flashes and night sweats: Many women experience hot flashes and night sweats during perimenopause. These sudden feelings of warmth or heat can be uncomfortable and disruptive.

Mood changes: Perimenopause can also cause mood changes, including irritability, anxiety, and depression.

Vaginal dryness: Declining estrogen levels can lead to vaginal dryness and discomfort during intercourse.

Sleep disturbances: Many women experience sleep disturbances during perimenopause, including difficulty falling asleep, waking up frequently during the night, and insomnia.

Decreased libido: Some women may experience a decrease in their sex drive or difficulty becoming aroused during perimenopause.

Changes in skin and hair: Perimenopause can also lead to changes in skin and hair, including dryness, thinning, and wrinkles.

Menopause

As a woman, menopause is a natural and inevitable part of life that we all eventually go through. Menopause marks the end of our reproductive years and is defined by the cessation of menstruation. This can be a significant milestone in our lives, as it marks the end of our ability to have children and signals a major shift in our bodies and hormones.

While menopause is a natural and normal process, it can also be challenging to navigate. Many women experience a range of physical and emotional symptoms during this time, including hot flashes, mood swings, vaginal dryness, and weight gain. These symptoms can be disruptive and uncomfortable, and can affect our quality of life.

In addition to physical symptoms, menopause can also bring up a range of emotions and feelings. It's common for women to experience a sense of loss or grief around the end of their reproductive years, and to struggle with feelings of anxiety, depression, or uncertainty about this new phase of life. However, it's important to remember that menopause is a natural and normal process, and that we can take steps to manage our symptoms and support our overall health and well-being.

Menopause is a significant milestone in a woman's life that can bring up a range of physical and emotional changes. While it can be challenging to navigate, there are several strategies and treatments available to help women manage their symptoms and support their health during this time. By taking care of ourselves and seeking support as needed, we can navigate this new phase of life with greater ease and comfort.

Postmenopause

Postmenopause is the stage of a woman's life that follows menopause, which is defined as the cessation of menstruation for a period of 12 consecutive months. During postmenopause, a woman's hormone levels stabilize at low levels, and she is no longer able to conceive.

Postmenopause is a normal and natural part of the aging process, and typically begins around the age of 50. During this time, women may experience a range of physical and emotional changes, including hot flashes, vaginal dryness, insomnia, and mood changes.

While the symptoms of postmenopause can be challenging, there are several strategies and treatments available to help women manage their symptoms and maintain their health during this time. Making dietary changes, such as reducing caffeine and alcohol intake, engaging in regular exercise, and getting enough sleep can all help to manage symptoms like hot flashes and mood changes.

Overall, postmenopause is a natural and normal part of a woman's life, and while it can be challenging to navigate, there are several strategies and treatments available to help women manage their symptoms and maintain their health during this time. By taking care of ourselves and seeking support as needed, we can navigate this new phase of life with greater ease and comfort.

The Galveston Diet and You

The Galveston Diet was specifically developed for women in midlife, particularly those going through perimenopause and menopause. As women age, their bodies undergo hormonal changes that can affect their metabolism and make it more difficult to lose weight or maintain a healthy weight. The Galveston Diet is designed to help women in midlife overcome these challenges and achieve optimal health.

The diet focuses on whole, nutrient-dense foods and emphasizes the importance of healthy fats and protein sources. It also incorporates intermittent fasting, which has been shown to improve insulin sensitivity and support healthy weight management.

In addition to its focus on nutrition and weight management, the Galveston Diet also incorporates lifestyle factors such as stress management, exercise, and sleep. These factors are particularly important for women in midlife, as they can help to manage symptoms like hot flashes, mood changes, and sleep disturbances.

HOW MIDDLE-AGED WOMEN CAN BENEFIT FROM THE GALVESTON DIET

Hormonal changes: As women go through perimenopause and menopause, their bodies undergo hormonal changes that can affect their metabolism and make it more difficult to maintain a healthy weight. The Galveston Diet is designed to support women in midlife by providing them with the nutrients and energy they need to support their changing bodies.

Nutrient-dense foods: The Galveston Diet focuses on whole, nutrient-dense foods that provide the body with the vitamins, minerals, and other nutrients it needs to function at its best. This can be especially important for women in midlife, who may be more susceptible to nutrient deficiencies.

Healthy fats and protein: The Galveston Diet emphasizes the importance of healthy fats and protein sources, which can help to support healthy hormone levels, improve insulin sensitivity, and promote satiety.

Intermittent fasting: The Galveston Diet incorporates intermittent fasting, which has been shown to support healthy weight management and improve insulin sensitivity. This can be especially important for women in midlife who may be struggling with weight gain and insulin resistance.

Stress management: The Galveston Diet emphasizes the importance of stress management, which can be especially important for women in midlife who may be dealing with increased stress levels related to work, family, and other responsibilities.

Exercise: The Galveston Diet encourages regular exercise, which can help to support healthy weight management, improve mood, and reduce the risk of chronic diseases.

Sleep: The Galveston Diet emphasizes the importance of getting enough sleep, which can be especially important for women in midlife who may be struggling with sleep disturbances related to perimenopause and menopause.

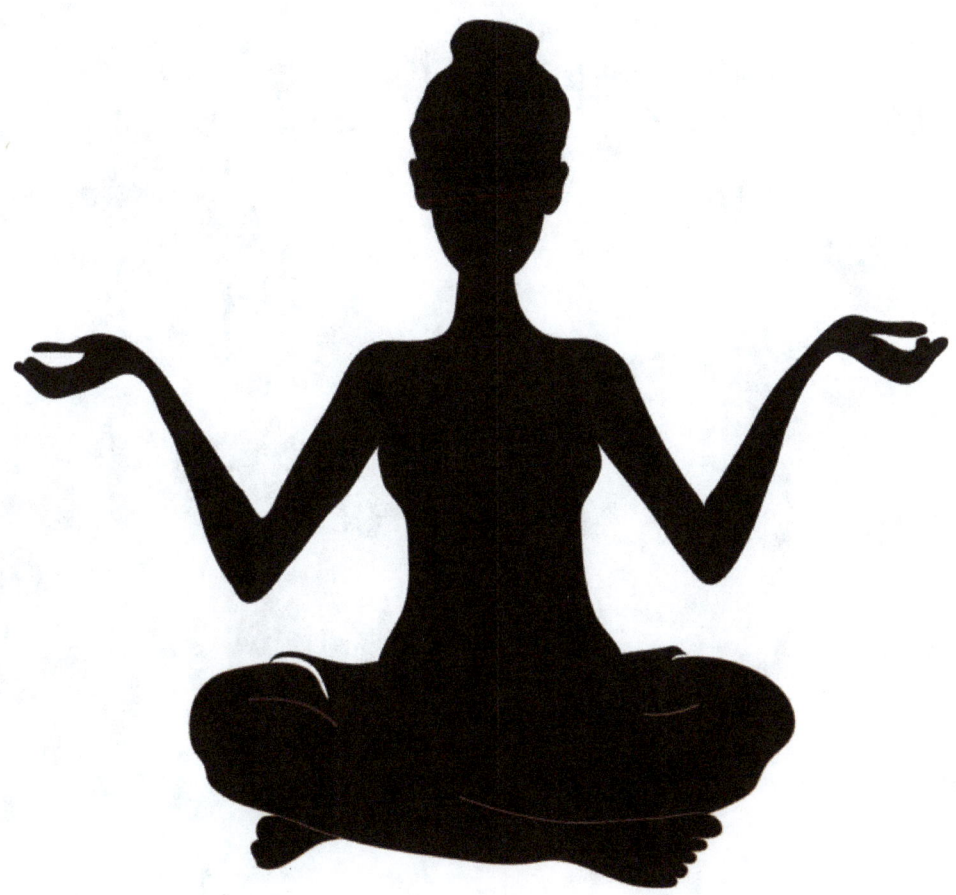

Chapter 2
Prepare to Change Your Life

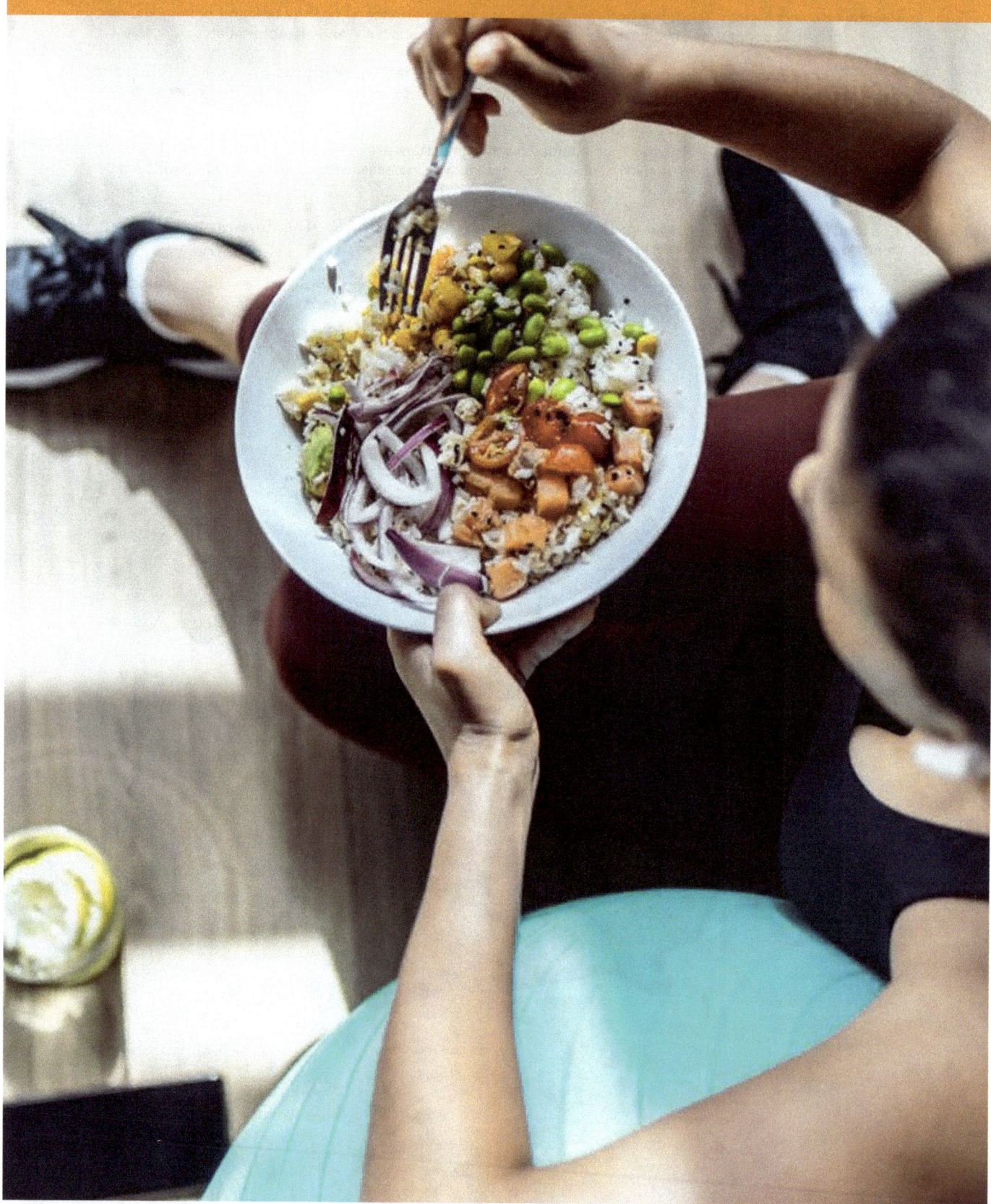

Know Your Measurements

Before starting the Galveston Diet, it's important for women to take certain bodily measurements and occasionally use a scale to gauge their results. This will help them track their progress and stay motivated as they work towards their weight loss and health goals.

Some of the important bodily measurements that women should take before starting the Galveston Diet include their weight, body mass index (BMI), waist circumference, and body fat percentage. By measuring these factors, women can get a better understanding of their current health status and track changes over time as they follow the Galveston Diet.

For example, monitoring changes in waist circumference can be a helpful way to track visceral fat, which is a type of fat that surrounds the internal organs and is associated with an increased risk of chronic diseases such as heart disease and diabetes. By tracking changes in waist circumference over time, women can see how their dietary and lifestyle changes are impacting their visceral fat levels and overall health.

In addition to taking bodily measurements, using a scale can also be a helpful tool for women on the Galveston Diet. While weight isn't the only factor that should be considered when tracking progress, it can be a useful way to monitor changes in body composition and overall health.

For example, a woman may not see significant changes in her weight on the scale, but she may notice that her clothes fit better or that she has more energy throughout the day. By using both bodily measurements and the scale to track progress, women can get a more comprehensive picture of how their bodies are changing over time.

Overall, taking bodily measurements and occasionally using a scale to gauge results is an important part of the Galveston Diet. By tracking progress and staying motivated, women can achieve their weight loss and health goals and improve their overall wellbeing.

Get a Nutrition Tracker

By monitoring their micronutrient and macronutrient intake, women can ensure that they're getting the right balance of nutrients to support their health and weight loss goals. For example, consuming adequate amounts of protein can help women feel fuller for longer periods of time, which can help with weight loss and weight management.

Similarly, tracking micronutrients such as iron, calcium, and vitamin D can help women maintain strong bones and prevent deficiencies that can impact overall health. It can also help women identify any nutrient gaps in their diet and make adjustments to ensure that they're getting all the nutrients their bodies need.

One way to monitor micronutrients and macronutrients is by using a food tracking app or journal. These tools can help women keep track of their food intake and make adjustments as needed to ensure they're getting the right balance of nutrients. Some apps and journals may also provide insights into the micronutrient and macronutrient content of certain foods, making it easier to plan meals that support optimal nutrition.

Overall, monitoring micronutrients and macronutrients can be an important component of success on the Galveston Diet. By ensuring that they're getting the right balance of nutrients, women can support their health and weight loss goals and optimize their overall wellbeing.

Start a Daily Journaling Practice

Set aside time each day: Start by setting aside a specific time each day to journal. This could be in the morning, during your lunch break, or in the evening. Choose a time that works best for you and commit to it.

Choose a format: Decide on the format you want to use for your journal. It could be a physical notebook, a digital document, or an app. Consider what format would be easiest and most enjoyable for you to use.

Write about your goals: Start by writing about your goals for following the Galveston Diet. What do you hope to achieve? What challenges do you anticipate? Writing about your goals can help you stay focused and motivated.

Track your progress: Use your journal to track your progress on the Galveston Diet. This could include tracking your food intake, your exercise routine, and your weight loss goals. Write about any successes or setbacks you experience along the way.

Reflect on your emotions: Use your journal as a space to reflect on your emotions and how they relate to your eating habits. Writing about your emotions can help you identify any triggers that may be impacting your eating patterns.

Celebrate your successes: Take time to celebrate your successes along the way. Write about your accomplishments and how they make you feel. Celebrating your successes can help you stay motivated and focused on your goals.

Remember, journaling is a personal practice, so there's no right or wrong way to do it. The most important thing is to find a format and approach that works best for you and helps you stay on track with your Galveston Diet journey.

Important Points to Note

Pregnant or breastfeeding women: The Galveston Diet is not recommended for pregnant or breastfeeding women, as their nutritional needs are different and require specific guidance from a healthcare provider.

Individuals with a history of eating disorders: Those who have a history of disordered eating, such as anorexia or bulimia, should approach any diet program with caution and seek guidance from a healthcare provider before starting.

People with certain medical conditions: Individuals with certain medical conditions, such as diabetes, heart disease, or kidney disease, should consult with a healthcare provider before starting the Galveston Diet to ensure it is safe and appropriate for their specific situation.

Those taking certain medications: Some medications may interact with the Galveston Diet or require adjustments in dosage, so it is important to discuss any medication use with a healthcare provider before starting the program.

Children: The Galveston Diet was designed specifically for women in perimenopause and menopause and is not recommended for children or adolescents, whose nutritional needs are different and require specific guidance from a healthcare provider.

Individuals with a history of yo-yo dieting: Those who have a history of yo-yo dieting or rapid weight loss and gain may need to approach any new diet program with caution and seek guidance from a healthcare provider before starting.

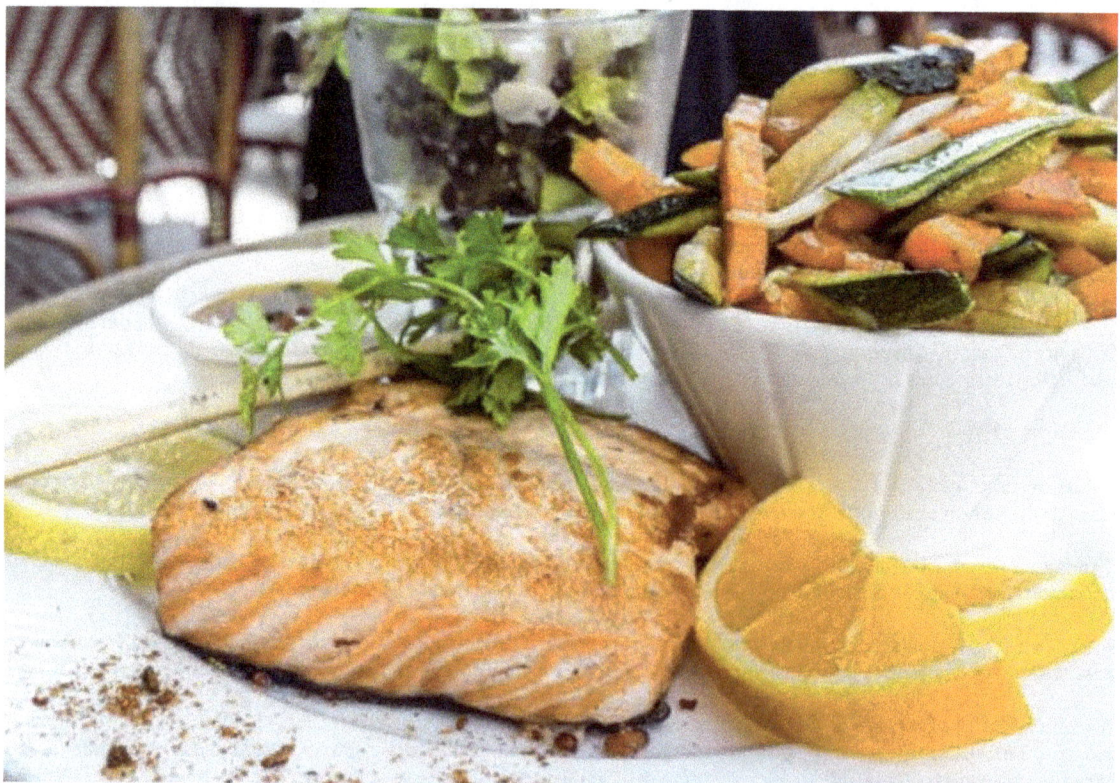

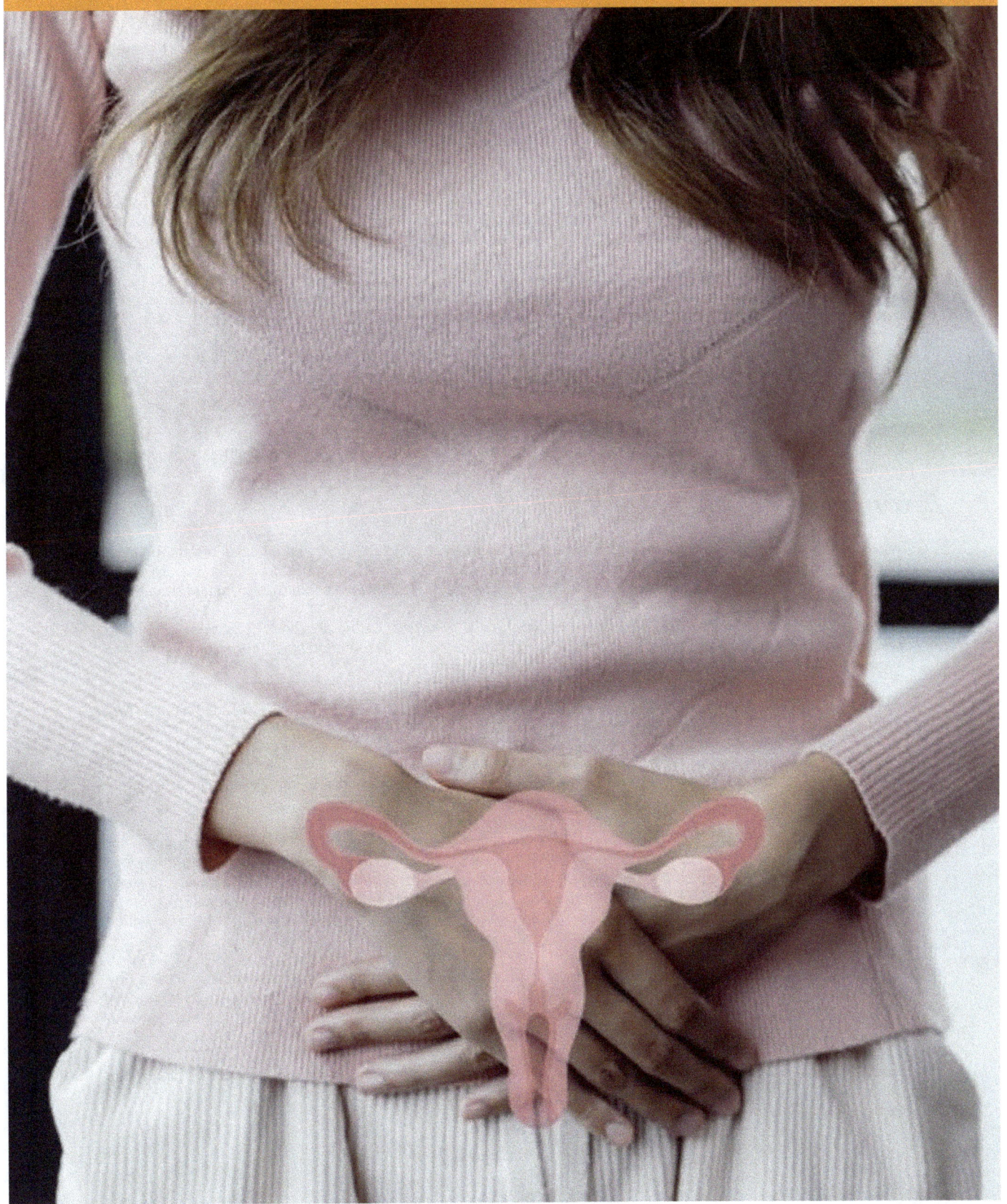

Action 1: Intermittent Fasting

Intermittent fasting is an eating pattern that involves alternating periods of eating with periods of fasting. The Galveston Diet incorporates intermittent fasting as one of its key strategies for weight loss and improved health. There are several different approaches to intermittent fasting, and the Galveston Diet recommends a 16:8 approach, which involves eating within an 8-hour window and fasting for the remaining 16 hours of the day.

Research has shown that intermittent fasting can have several health benefits. For example, a 2019 study published in the New England Journal of Medicine found that intermittent fasting can improve blood pressure, insulin sensitivity, and cholesterol levels. Another study published in the Journal of the Academy of Nutrition and Dietetics found that intermittent fasting can lead to weight loss and improved body composition.

In addition to these benefits, intermittent fasting can also be an effective tool for weight loss. For example, a study published in the journal Obesity Reviews found that intermittent fasting can lead to greater weight loss than traditional calorie restriction diets.

To incorporate intermittent fasting into the Galveston Diet, individuals can follow the 16:8 approach, which involves eating within an 8-hour window and fasting for the remaining 16 hours of the day. For example, someone following this approach might eat their first meal at 12 pm and their last meal at 8 pm, then fast until 12 pm the following day.

During the eating window, individuals should focus on nutrient-dense foods, such as fresh vegetables and fruits, lean protein sources, healthy fats, and complex carbohydrates. It's also important to stay hydrated and drink plenty of water throughout the day.

It's important to note that intermittent fasting may not be appropriate for everyone. Pregnant or breastfeeding women, individuals with a history of disordered eating, and those with certain medical conditions should consult with a healthcare provider before trying intermittent fasting or any new diet or weight loss program.

Overall, the Galveston Diet's incorporation of intermittent fasting can be a helpful tool for weight loss and improved health. However, it's important to follow the approach safely and under the guidance of a healthcare provider or registered dietitian.

TYPES OF FASTING

Time-Restricted Feeding: This is the most common type of intermittent fasting, which involves restricting your daily eating window to a specific period of time, such as 8 hours. The remaining 16 hours of the day are spent fasting. Time-restricted feeding has been shown to improve weight loss, metabolic health, and insulin sensitivity.

Alternate-Day Fasting: This involves alternating between days of normal eating and days of fasting. On fasting days, you consume only a small amount of calories or no calories at all. Alternate-day fasting has been shown to improve weight loss, reduce inflammation, and improve heart health.

5:2 Diet: This involves eating normally for five days of the week and then restricting calories to around 500-600 on two non-consecutive days. The 5:2 diet has been shown to improve weight loss, reduce inflammation, and improve insulin sensitivity.

Eat-Stop-Eat: This involves fasting for 24 hours once or twice a week. On fasting days, you consume no calories at all. Eat-stop-eat has been shown to improve weight loss, reduce inflammation, and improve insulin sensitivity.

Action 2: Anti-Inflammatory Nutrition

Anti-inflammatory nutrition is an eating pattern that focuses on consuming foods that have been shown to reduce inflammation in the body. The Galveston Diet incorporates anti-inflammatory nutrition as a key strategy for weight loss and improved health. There is growing evidence that chronic inflammation is linked to a range of health problems, including heart disease, cancer, and obesity. Anti-inflammatory nutrition can help to reduce inflammation and promote better health.

Research has shown that anti-inflammatory foods can have several health benefits. For example, a 2019 study published in the American Journal of Clinical Nutrition found that consuming a diet high in anti-inflammatory foods can reduce the risk of heart disease. Another study published in the Journal of the Academy of Nutrition and Dietetics found that anti-inflammatory diets can lead to weight loss and improved body composition.

To incorporate anti-inflammatory nutrition into the Galveston Diet, individuals should focus on consuming foods that are rich in anti-inflammatory compounds, such as fruits, vegetables, whole grains, lean protein sources, healthy fats, and spices. For example, foods like berries, leafy greens, fatty fish, nuts, and turmeric all have anti-inflammatory properties.

It's also important to avoid or limit foods that are known to promote inflammation, such as processed foods, sugary drinks, and foods high in saturated fats or trans fats. For example, instead of choosing processed snacks or sugary desserts, individuals on the Galveston Diet may opt for fresh fruit or a small serving of dark chocolate as a treat.

In addition to reducing inflammation, consuming a diet that is high in anti-inflammatory foods can also support weight loss and improved overall health. By focusing on whole, nutrient-dense foods and limiting highly processed and inflammatory foods, individuals can improve their body composition, reduce their risk of chronic disease, and increase their overall vitality.

It's important to note that anti-inflammatory nutrition is not a cure-all and should be used in conjunction with other healthy lifestyle practices, such as regular exercise and stress management. Additionally, individuals should consult with a healthcare provider or registered dietitian before starting any new diet or weight loss program.

Action 3: Fuel Refocus

The Fuel Refocus strategy is an important part of the Galveston Diet that can help women shift their focus away from counting calories and towards consuming nutritious foods that provide sustained energy throughout the day. By emphasizing the importance of consuming foods that are high in protein, healthy fats, and fiber, while limiting processed and sugary foods, the Fuel Refocus strategy can help women achieve their weight loss goals and improve their overall health.

Research has shown that consuming a diet that is high in protein and fiber can lead to greater weight loss and improved body composition in women. For example, a 2015 study published in the American Journal of Clinical Nutrition found that a high-protein diet can lead to greater weight loss and fat loss in women compared to a low-protein diet.

To implement the Fuel Refocus strategy on the Galveston Diet, women should focus on consuming foods that provide sustained energy throughout the day. This includes foods such as lean protein sources like chicken, fish, and tofu, healthy fats like avocado, nuts, and olive oil, and high-fiber carbohydrates like whole grains, fruits, and vegetables.

A typical Fuel Refocus meal on the Galveston Diet for women might be a salad with grilled chicken, avocado, and mixed greens, or grilled salmon with a side of roasted vegetables and quinoa. By focusing on nutrient-dense, high-quality foods, women on the Galveston Diet can improve their energy levels, support weight loss, and improve their overall health.

It's important to remember that the Fuel Refocus strategy is just one component of a healthy lifestyle, and women should also incorporate other healthy habits into their daily routine, such as regular exercise and stress management. Before starting any new diet or weight loss program, it's important for women to consult with a healthcare provider or registered dietitian to ensure it's safe and appropriate for their individual needs.

The Galveston Diet is a nutrition program designed specifically for women in perimenopause and menopause to help them lose weight and improve their overall health and wellness.

Q&A

What are some of the key foods to eat on the Galveston Diet?
The Galveston Diet emphasizes whole, nutrient-dense foods such as fruits, vegetables, lean proteins, and healthy fats. Some specific examples include leafy greens, berries, nuts, seeds, salmon, avocado, and olive oil.

Can I still eat carbohydrates on the Galveston Diet?
Yes, the Galveston Diet does not require complete elimination of carbohydrates. However, the diet emphasizes choosing complex carbohydrates over refined ones, such as whole grains instead of white bread or pasta.
How long does it take to see results on the Galveston Diet?

Results can vary depending on individual factors such as starting weight and overall health status, but many women report seeing improvements in energy levels and weight loss within the first few weeks of starting the program.

Do I need to exercise while following the Galveston Diet?
While exercise is not strictly required, incorporating some form of physical activity can help enhance the results of the Galveston Diet and improve overall health and wellness. The Galveston Diet recommends aiming for at least 30 minutes of moderate exercise most days of the week.

Chapter 4
The Meal Plans and Shopping Lists

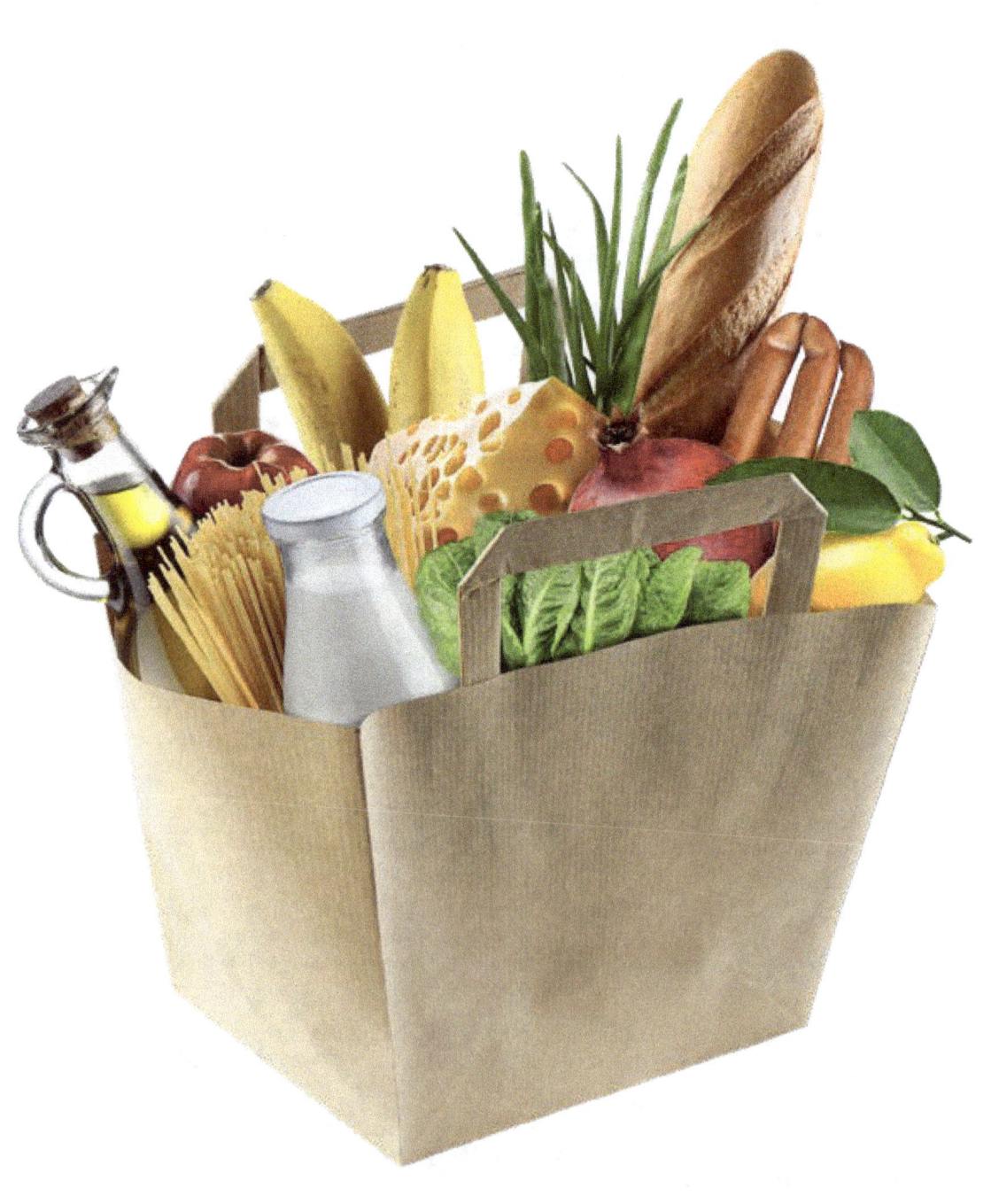

The Conventional Menus: Week 1

Day 1

Meal 1: Slow-Cooker Vegan Split Pea Soup
Snack 1: Coconut Citrus Tart
Meal 2: Asian-Inspired Salmon
Snack 2: Coconut Citrus Tart
Macros: Fat:38, Protein:35.8, Net Carbs:35.8, Fiber:6.8

Day 2

Meal 1: Slow-Cooker Vegan Split Pea Soup
Snack 1: Coconut Citrus Tart
Meal 2: Asian-Inspired Salmon
Snack 2: Coconut Citrus Tart
Macros: Fat:38, Protein:35.8, Net Carbs:35.8, Fiber:6.8

Day 3

Meal 1: Slow-Cooker Vegan Split Pea Soup
Snack 1: Coconut Citrus Tart
Meal 2: Asian-Inspired Salmon
Snack 2: Coconut Citrus Tart
Macros: Fat:38, Protein:35.8, Net Carbs:35.8, Fiber:6.8

Day 4

Meal 1: Slow-Cooker Vegan Split Pea Soup
Snack 1: Coconut Citrus Tart
Meal 2: Asian-Inspired Salmon
Snack 2: Coconut Citrus Tart
Macros: Fat:38, Protein:35.8, Net Carbs:35.8, Fiber:6.8

Day 5

Meal 1: Slow-Cooker Vegan Split Pea Soup
Snack 1: Coconut Citrus Tart
Meal 2: Turkey Larb Lettuce Wraps
Snack 2: Coconut Citrus Tart
Macros: Fat:29, Protein:29.8, Net Carbs:29.8, Fiber:5.8

Day 6

Meal 1: Slow-Cooker Vegan Split Pea Soup
Snack 1: Coconut Citrus Tart
Meal 2: Turkey Larb Lettuce Wraps
Snack 2: Coconut Citrus Tart
Macros: Fat:29, Protein:29.8, Net Carbs:29.8, Fiber:5.8

Day 7

Meal 1: Slow-Cooker Vegan Split Pea Soup
Snack 1: Coconut Citrus Tart
Meal 2: Turkey Larb Lettuce Wraps
Snack 2: Coconut Citrus Tart
Macros: Fat:29, Protein:29.8, Net Carbs:29.8, Fiber:5.8

Shopping List for Week 1

Note: Amounts given here indicate the quantities you need for the week's recipes; they are not always indicative of the quantities in which the items are commonly sold.

Vegetables:
- 2 small sweet potatoes
- 1 small red onion
- 4 scallions
- Romaine lettuce leaves

Fruits:
- 1 lime or lemon

Proteins
- 2.5 cups green or yellow split peas
- 4 salmon fillets
- 1 pound ground turkey

Nuts:
- 2 tablespoons unsweetened shredded coconut

Miscellaneous :
- 1 tablespoon dried thyme
- 1½ teaspoons salt
- 3 tbsp miso paste
- 1 tsp coconut aminos
- 2 tablespoons freshly squeezed lime juice
- 2 tablespoons fish sauce
- 2 tablespoons minced fresh cilantro
- 1 tablespoon minced fresh mint (optional)
- 1 tablespoon coconut sugar
- 2 tablespoons granulated erythritol or other low-carb sweetener
- 1 (13.5-ounce) can full-fat coconut milk
- 2 tablespoons ghee, unsalted butter, or lard
- 1 teaspoon pure vanilla extract
- Pinch of fine Himalayan salt
- 1 tablespoon unflavored grass-fed beef gelatin
- 1 Pie Crust

The Conventional Menus: Week 2

Day 1

Meal 1: Blueberry-Millet Breakfast Bake
Snack 1: Homemade Trail Mix
Meal 2: Spaghetti Bolognese
Snack 2: Avocado Fudge
Macros: Fat:45, Protein:26, Net Carbs:126, Fiber:14

Day 2

Meal 1: Blueberry-Millet Breakfast Bake
Snack 1: Homemade Trail Mix
Meal 2: Spaghetti Bolognese
Snack 2: Avocado Fudge
Macros: Fat:45, Protein:26, Net Carbs:126, Fiber:14

Day 3

Meal 1: Blueberry-Millet Breakfast Bake
Snack 1: Homemade Trail Mix
Meal 2: Spaghetti Bolognese
Snack 2: Avocado Fudge
Macros: Fat:45, Protein:26, Net Carbs:126, Fiber:14

Day 4

Meal 1: Blueberry-Millet Breakfast Bake
Snack 1: Homemade Trail Mix
Meal 2: Spaghetti Bolognese
Snack 2: Avocado Fudge
Macros: Fat:45, Protein:26, Net Carbs:126, Fiber:14

Day 5

Meal 1: Blueberry-Millet Breakfast Bake
Snack 1: Homemade Trail Mix
Meal 2: Spaghetti Bolognese
Snack 2: Avocado Fudge
Macros: Fat:45, Protein:26, Net Carbs:126, Fiber:14

Day 6

Meal 1: Blueberry-Millet Breakfast Bake
Snack 1: Homemade Trail Mix
Meal 2: Spaghetti Bolognese
Snack 2: Avocado Fudge
Macros: Fat:45, Protein:26, Net Carbs:126, Fiber:14

Day 7

Meal 1: Blueberry-Millet Breakfast Bake
Snack 1: Homemade Trail Mix
Meal 2: Spaghetti Bolognese
Snack 2: Avocado Fudge
Macros: Fat:45, Protein:26, Net Carbs:126, Fiber:14

Shopping List for Week 2

Vegetables:
- 3 garlic cloves
- 1/2 cup chopped white onion
- 2/3 cup chopped celery
- 2/3 cup chopped carrot

Fruits:
- 2 cups fresh or frozen blueberries
- 1 cup raisins
- 1 cup dried cranberries
- 1 ripe avocado

Nuts:
- 1 cup pumpkin seeds
- 1 cup sunflower seeds
- 1 cup large coconut flakes
- Optional: 1/2 cup cacao nibs

Proteins:
- 1 pound lean ground beef

Miscellaneous:
- 2 cups millet
- 1 3/4 cups unsweetened applesauce
- 1/3 cup + 1/4 cup coconut oil
- 2 teaspoons grated fresh ginger
- 1 1/2 teaspoons ground cinnamon
- 1 1/2 cups bittersweet chocolate chips
- 1 tablespoon white wine vinegar
- 1/2 teaspoon red pepper flakes
- 1/8 teaspoon ground nutmeg
- 1/2 teaspoon sea salt

The Conventional Menus: Week 3

Day 1

Meal 1: Mini Quiche Muffins
Snack 1: Chewy Chocolate Chip Cookies
Meal 2: Baked Scotch Eggs
Snack 2: Banana "Nice" Cream
Macros: Fat:36, Protein:27.6, Net Carbs: 90.3, Fiber:11.5

Day 2

Meal 1: Mini Quiche Muffins
Snack 1: Chewy Chocolate Chip Cookies
Meal 2: Baked Scotch Eggs
Snack 2: Banana "Nice" Cream
Macros: Fat:36, Protein:27.6, Net Carbs: 90.3, Fiber:11.5

Day 3

Meal 1: Mini Quiche Muffins
Snack 1: Chewy Chocolate Chip Cookies
Meal 2: Baked Scotch Eggs
Snack 2: Banana "Nice" Cream
Macros: Fat:36, Protein:27.6, Net Carbs: 90.3, Fiber:11.5

Day 4

Meal 1: Mini Quiche Muffins
Snack 1: Chewy Chocolate Chip Cookies
Meal 2: Baked Scotch Eggs
Snack 2: Banana "Nice" Cream
Macros: Fat:36, Protein:27.6, Net Carbs: 90.3, Fiber:11.5

Day 5

Meal 1: Mini Quiche Muffins
Snack 1: Chewy Chocolate Chip Cookies
Meal 2: Baked Scotch Eggs
Snack 2: Banana "Nice" Cream
Macros: Fat:36, Protein:27.6, Net Carbs: 90.3, Fiber:11.5

Day 6

Meal 1: Mini Quiche Muffins
Snack 1: Chewy Chocolate Chip Cookies
Meal 2: Baked Scotch Eggs
Snack 2: Banana "Nice" Cream
Macros: Fat:36, Protein:27.6, Net Carbs: 90.3, Fiber:11.5

Day 7

Meal 1: Mini Quiche Muffins
Snack 1: Chewy Chocolate Chip Cookies
Meal 2: Baked Scotch Eggs
Snack 2: Banana "Nice" Cream
Macros: Fat:36, Protein:27.6, Net Carbs: 90.3, Fiber:11.5

Shopping List for Week 3

Vegetables:
• 2 cups Rainbow slaw
• 4 frozen Bananas, diced

Proteins:
• 4 slices Bacon
• 13 Large eggs
• Ground pork sausage (enough for 8 servings)
• 1 tablespoon Beef gelatin

Nuts and Seeds:
• 2 tablespoons shelled hemp seeds (optional)

Dairy and Dairy Substitutes:
• 1/2 cup Full-fat coconut milk
• 1/4 cup Unsweetened butter
• 1/4 cup Ghee or clarified butter
• 1 (4-ounce) bar or 1/2 cup Stevia-sweetened semisweet baking chocolate

Flours and Baking Ingredients:
• 5/8 cup Coconut flour
• 4 to 5 tablespoons Flaxseed meal
• 1 tablespoon Unflavored grass-fed beef gelatin
• 1/2 teaspoon Baking soda

Miscellaneous:
• 1/3 cup Granulated erythritol or other low-carb sweetener
• 1/4 cup Nutritional yeast
• 3 teaspoons Himalayan salt
• 2 tablespoons Avocado oil
• 1 to 3 tablespoons Ice-cold water

The Conventional Menus: Week 4

Day 1

Meal 1: Chilled Coconut-Avocado Soup
Snack 1: Hot Cashew Hummus
Meal 2: Open-Face Avocado Tuna Melts
Snack 2: Coconut-Mango Lassi
Macros: Fat: 101, Protein:42, Net Carbs:82, Fiber17

Day 2

Meal 1: Chilled Coconut-Avocado Soup
Snack 1: Hot Cashew Hummus
Meal 2: Open-Face Avocado Tuna Melts
Snack 2: Coconut-Mango Lassi
Macros: Fat: 101, Protein:42, Net Carbs:82, Fiber17

Day 3

Meal 1: Chilled Coconut-Avocado Soup
Snack 1: Hot Cashew Hummus
Meal 2: Open-Face Avocado Tuna Melts
Snack 2: Coconut-Mango Lassi
Macros: Fat: 101, Protein:42, Net Carbs:82, Fiber17

Day 4

Meal 1: Chilled Coconut-Avocado Soup
Snack 1: Hot Cashew Hummus
Meal 2: Open-Face Avocado Tuna Melts
Snack 2: Coconut-Mango Lassi
Macros: Fat: 101, Protein:42, Net Carbs:82, Fiber17

Day 5

Meal 1: Chilled Coconut-Avocado Soup
Snack 1: Hot Cashew Hummus
Meal 2: Open-Face Avocado Tuna Melts
Snack 2: Coconut-Mango Lassi
Macros: Fat: 101, Protein:42, Net Carbs:82, Fiber17

Day 6

Meal 1: Chilled Coconut-Avocado Soup
Snack 1: Hot Cashew Hummus
Meal 2: Open-Face Avocado Tuna Melts
Snack 2: Coconut-Mango Lassi
Macros: Fat: 101, Protein:42, Net Carbs:82, Fiber17

Day 7

Meal 1: Chilled Coconut-Avocado Soup
Snack 1: Hot Cashew Hummus
Meal 2: Open-Face Avocado Tuna Melts
Snack 2: Coconut-Mango Lassi
Macros: Fat: 101, Protein:42, Net Carbs:82, Fiber17

Shopping List for Week 4

Vegetables:
- 1/4 cup Chopped red onion

Fruits:
- 3 Ripe avocado, peeled and pitted
- 2 Freshly squeezed lemon juice
- 1 1/2 cups Frozen mango chunks
- 1 Tomato, cut into 8 slices

Nuts:
- 1 cup Raw cashews

Proteins:
- 2 (5-ounce) cans Wild-caught albacore tuna
- 1/4 cup Shredded raw Parmesan cheese, divided

Miscellaneous :
- 1 cup Herbed Chicken Bone Broth
- 2 cups Canned full-fat coconut milk
- 1/4 cup Paleo mayonnaise
- 2 Crushed garlic cloves
- 1 tbsp Extra-virgin olive oil
- 1/2 cup Plain yogurt
- 1 tbsp Honey
- Sea salt, to taste
- Freshly ground black pepper, to taste
- Fresh dill, chopped, 1/2 tsp + fresh dill sprigs for garnish
- 1 tbsp Fresh ginger, grated
- 1/4 tsp Cayenne pepper
- Ground cardamom, pinch
- Sourdough bread
- Paprika, to taste
- 2 tbsp Minced shallot
- 1 cup Ice cubes

The Vegetarian Menus: Week1

Day 1

Meal 1: Carrot-Ginger Soup
Snack 1: Butternut Squash Fries
Meal 2: Balsamic Beets
Snack 2: Roasted Apricots
Macros: Fat:34, Protein:8, Net Carbs:89, Fiber:15

Day 2

Meal 1: Carrot-Ginger Soup
Snack 1: Butternut Squash Fries
Meal 2: Balsamic Beets
Snack 2: Roasted Apricots
Macros: Fat:34, Protein:8, Net Carbs:89, Fiber:15

Day 3

Meal 1: Carrot-Ginger Soup
Snack 1: Butternut Squash Fries
Meal 2: Balsamic Beets
Snack 2: Roasted Apricots
Macros: Fat:34, Protein:8, Net Carbs:89, Fiber:15

Day 4

Meal 1: Carrot-Ginger Soup
Snack 1: Butternut Squash Fries
Meal 2: Balsamic Beets
Snack 2: Roasted Apricots
Macros: Fat:34, Protein:8, Net Carbs:89, Fiber:15

Day 5

Meal 1: Carrot-Ginger Soup
Snack 1: Butternut Squash Fries
Meal 2: Balsamic Beets
Snack 2: Roasted Apricots
Macros: Fat:34, Protein:8, Net Carbs:89, Fiber:15

Day 6

Meal 1: Carrot-Ginger Soup
Snack 1: Butternut Squash Fries
Meal 2: Balsamic Beets
Snack 2: Roasted Apricots
Macros: Fat:34, Protein:8, Net Carbs:89, Fiber:15

Day 7

Meal 1: Carrot-Ginger Soup
Snack 1: Butternut Squash Fries
Meal 2: Balsamic Beets
Snack 2: Roasted Apricots
Macros: Fat:34, Protein:8, Net Carbs:89, Fiber:15

Shopping List for Vegetarian Week 1

Vegetables:
- 8 carrots
- 1 large onion
- 4 to 6 medium beets
- 1 large butternut squash
- 20 fresh apricots

Fruits:
- 20 fresh apricots
- 1 cup apple juice

Miscellaneous:
- 2 cups unsweetened coconut milk
- 2 tablespoons coconut oil
- ¼ cup balsamic vinegar
- 1.5-inch piece fresh ginger
- 3 fresh rosemary sprigs
- Cardamom (optional)

- Sea salt
- Black pepper
- Garlic powder
- Balsamic vinegar

The Vegetarian Menus: Week 2

Day 1

Meal 1: Wild Mushroom Frittata
Snack 1: Spicy Mixed Nuts
Meal 2: Green Pasta Salad
Snack 2: Mixed Bean Dip
Macros: Fat:45.5, Protein:43, Net Carbs:119, Fiber:41

Day 2

Meal 1: Wild Mushroom Frittata
Snack 1: Spicy Mixed Nuts
Meal 2: Green Pasta Salad
Snack 2: Mixed Bean Dip
Macros: Fat:45.5, Protein:43, Net Carbs:119, Fiber:41

Day 3

Meal 1: Wild Mushroom Frittata
Snack 1: Spicy Mixed Nuts
Meal 2: Green Pasta Salad
Snack 2: Mixed Bean Dip
Macros: Fat:45.5, Protein:43, Net Carbs:119, Fiber:41

Day 4

Meal 1: Wild Mushroom Frittata
Snack 1: Spicy Mixed Nuts
Meal 2: Green Pasta Salad
Snack 2: Mixed Bean Dip
Macros: Fat:45.5, Protein:43, Net Carbs:119, Fiber:41

Day 5

Meal 1: Wild Mushroom Frittata
Snack 1: Spicy Mixed Nuts
Meal 2: Green Pasta Salad
Snack 2: Mixed Bean Dip
Macros: Fat:45.5, Protein:43, Net Carbs:119, Fiber:41

Day 6

Meal 1: Wild Mushroom Frittata
Snack 1: Spicy Mixed Nuts
Meal 2: Green Pasta Salad
Snack 2: Mixed Bean Dip
Macros: Fat:45.5, Protein:43, Net Carbs:119, Fiber:41

Day 7

Meal 1: Wild Mushroom Frittata
Snack 1: Spicy Mixed Nuts
Meal 2: Green Pasta Salad
Snack 2: Mixed Bean Dip
Macros: Fat:45.5, Protein:43, Net Carbs:119, Fiber:41

Shopping List for Vegetarian Week 2

Vegetables:
- 2 cups sliced wild mushrooms
- 1/2 sweet onion
- 1 bunch asparagus
- 2 cups arugula
- 2 scallions
- 2 cherry tomatoes

Nuts:
- 1 cup almonds
- 1/2 cup walnuts
- 1/4 cup sunflower seeds

Miscellaneous:
- 1/2 cup unsweetened almond milk
- 1 (12-ounce) package gluten-free penne or fusilli
- 1 tablespoon olive oil
- 1 teaspoon ground cumin
- 1/2 teaspoon ground coriander
- 2 teaspoons bottled minced garlic
- 1 tablespoon chopped fresh oregano
- 1 tsp ground turmeric
- 1/4 cup pumpkin puree
- 1 tbsp apple cider vinegar
- 2 tsp honey
- 1 tsp lime juice
- Sea salt
- Black pepper
- Garlic powder
- Red pepper flakes
- Cayenne pepper

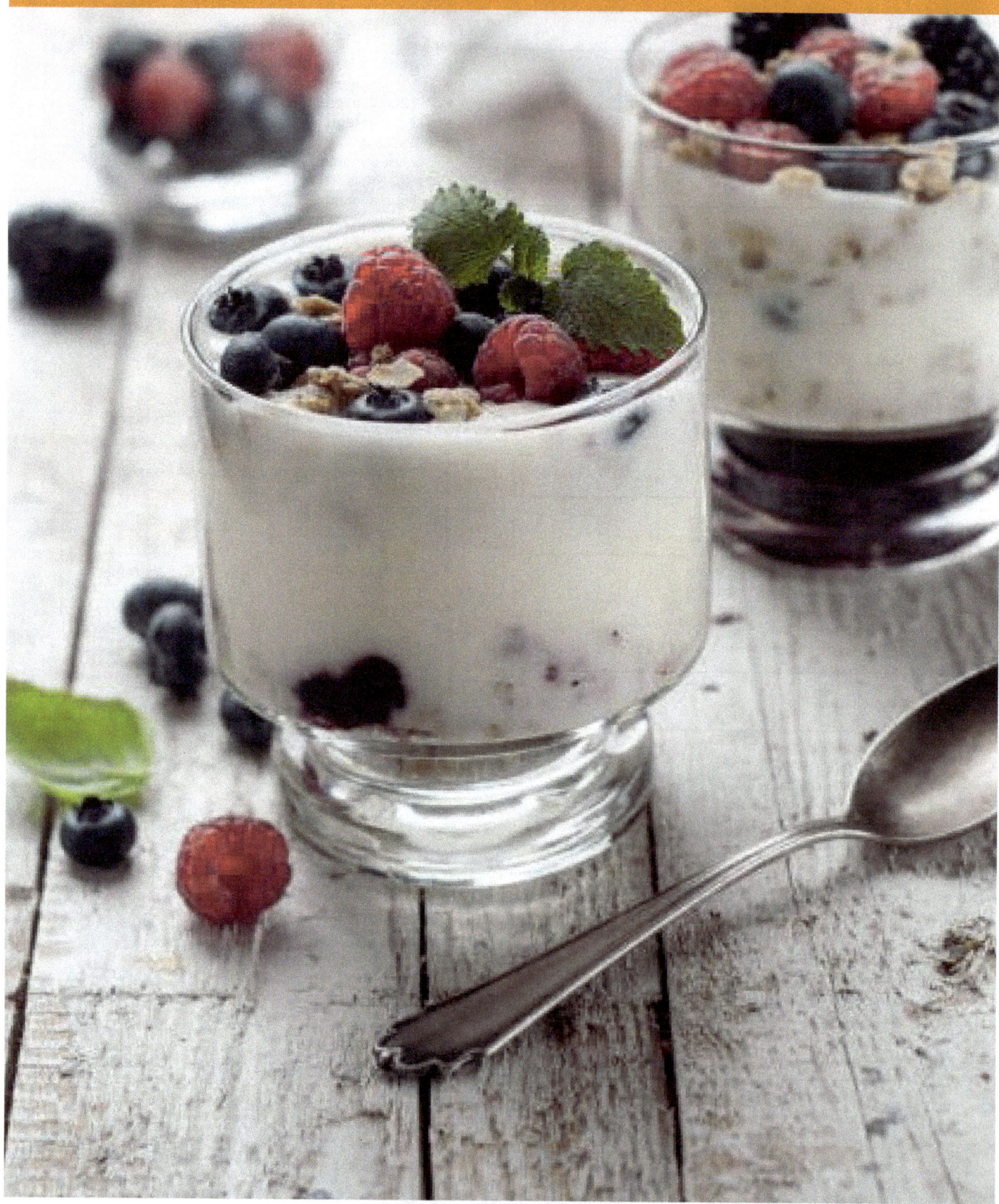

Chapter 5
Smoothies & Breakfast

Chai Smoothie

Prep time: 5 minutes|Cooking time:10 minutes|Serves 2

- 1 cup unsweetened almond milk
- 1 cup pure pumpkin purée
- 1 tablespoon pure maple syrup
- 1 teaspoon grated fresh peeled ginger
- ¼ teaspoon ground cinnamon
- ⅛ teaspoon ground nutmeg
- Pinch ground cloves
- Pinch ground cardamom
- 4 ice cubes

1. In a blender, combine the almond milk, pumpkin, maple syrup, ginger, cinnamon, nutmeg, cloves, and cardamom. Blend until smooth.
2. Add the ice and blend until thick.

PER SERVING

Calories 88| Total fat 2g| Saturated fat 0g| Carbohydrates 18g| Fiber 4g| Protein 2g

Sour Cherry & Pumpkin Seed Granola

Prep time: 10 minutes|Cooking time:5 to 6 hours |Serves 4 to 6

- 5 tablespoons melted coconut oil, divided
- 1 cup unsweetened shredded coconut
- 1 cup rolled oats
- 1 cup pecans
- ½ cup pumpkin seeds
- 1 ripe banana
- 1 tablespoon vanilla extract
- ½ teaspoon sea salt
- ½ teaspoon ground cinnamon
- ½ teaspoon ground ginger
- 1 cup dried sour cherries

1. Coat the slow cooker with 1 tablespoon of coconut oil.
2. In your slow cooker, toss together the coconut, oats, pecans, and pumpkin seeds.
3. In a small bowl, mash the banana with the remaining ¼ cup of melted coconut oil, the vanilla, salt, cinnamon, and ginger.
4. Add the liquid ingredients to the granola mixture and stir well to combine.
5. Cover the cooker and set to low. Cook for 5 to 6 hours (see Tip).
6. When the cooking is finished, stir in the cherries.
7. Spread the granola on a flat surface or baking sheet to cool and dry completely before storing in airtight containers.
8. Stored in a cool place, this will keep up to six months.

PER SERVING

Calories 777| Total Fat 58g| Total Carbs 58g| Sugar 25g| Fiber 10g| Protein 7g| Sodium 306mg

Morning Millet

Prep time: 15 minutes|Cooking time:7 to 8 hours|Serves 4

- 1 cup millet
- 2 cups water
- 2 cups full-fat coconut milk
- ½ teaspoon sea salt
- ½ teaspoon ground cinnamon
- ½ teaspoon ground ginger
- ¼ teaspoon vanilla extract
- ½ cup fresh blueberries

1. In your slow cooker, combine the millet, water, coconut milk, salt, cinnamon, ginger, and vanilla. Stir well.
2. Cover the cooker and set to low. Cook for 7 to 8 hours.
3. Stir in the blueberries to warm at the end and serve.

PER SERVING

Calories 276| Total Fat 22g| Total Carbs 18g| Sugar 3g| Fiber 1g| Protein 3g| Sodium 323mg

Caramel-Apple Oats

Prep time: 15 minutes|Cooking time:6 to 8 hours |Serves 4

- 1 tablespoon coconut oil
- 3 sweet apples, such as Fuji or Gala, peeled and sliced
- 2 tablespoons coconut sugar
- ¼ teaspoon sea salt
- 1 teaspoon ground ginger
- 1 teaspoon ground cinnamon
- 1 teaspoon vanilla extract
- 2 cups rolled oats
- 1 cup unsweetened applesauce
- 3 cups unsweetened almond milk
- ½ cup water

1. Coat the slow cooker with the coconut oil.
2. Layer the sliced apples along the bottom of the slow cooker so each piece is touching the bottom.
3. In this order, layer in the coconut sugar, salt, ginger, cinnamon, vanilla, oats, applesauce, almond milk, and water.
4. Cover the cooker and set to low. Cook for 6 to 8 hours and serve.

PER SERVING

Calories 313| Total Fat 9g| Total Carbs 56g| Sugar 24g| Fiber 8g| Protein 6g| Sodium 274mg

"Chocolate"-Avocado Smoothie

Prep time: 5 minutes|Cooking time:10 minutes|Serves 2

- 1 cup unsweetened almond milk
- 1 cup shredded kale
- ½ avocado
- ½ banana
- 2 tablespoons carob powder
- 1 tablespoon coconut oil
- 1 tablespoon raw honey
- 1 teaspoon pure vanilla extract
- 4 ice cubes

1. In a blender, combine the almond milk, kale, avocado, banana, carob powder, coconut oil, honey, and vanilla. Blend until smooth.
2. Add the ice and blend until thick.

PER SERVING

Calories 295| Total fat 19g| Saturated fat 10g| Carbohydrates 27g| Fiber 5g| Protein 3g

Mango Green Tea Smoothie

Prep time: 5 minutes|Cooking time:10 minutes|Serves 2

- 1 tbsp fresh mint, chopped
- 2 cups mango, cubed
- 2 tsp turmeric powder
- 2 tbsp green tea powder
- 2 cups almond milk
- 2 tbsp honey
- 1 cup crushed ice

1. Place the mint, mango, turmeric, green tea, almond milk, honey, and ice in a blender and pulse until smooth. Serve.

PER SERVING

Cal 290| Fat 4g| Carbs 69g| Protein 5g

Blueberry Smoothie with Ginger

Prep time: 5 minutes|Cooking time:10 minutes|Serves 2

- 1 cup fresh blueberries
- 2 cups almond milk
- 1 (0.07-oz) packet stevia
- 2 cups crushed ice
- in piece fresh ginger, peeled and chopped

1. Place the blueberries, almond milk, stevia, ginger, and ice in a blender and pulse until smooth. Serve right away.

PER SERVING

Cal 96| Fat 4g| Carbs 17g| Protein 4g

Morning Matcha & Ginger Shake

Prep time: 5 minutes|Cooking time:10 minutes|Serves 2

- 1 tbsp hemp seeds
- 1 tbsp grated ginger
- 2 tbsp honey
- 2 tbsp matcha powder
- 2 cups almond milk
- 1 cup ice

1. Place the hemp seeds, ginger, honey, matcha, ice, and milk in a blender and pulse until smooth. Serve.

PER SERVING

Cal 350| Fat 8g| Carbs 57g| Protein 10g

Minty Green Smoothie

Prep time: 5 minutes|Cooking time:10 minutes|Serves 2

- 1 cup canned lite coconut milk
- 1 cup fresh spinach
- 1 banana, cut into chunks
- ½ avocado
- ½ English cucumber, cut into chunks
- 2 tablespoons chopped fresh mint
- 1 tablespoon freshly squeezed lemon juice
- 1 tablespoon raw honey
- 3 ice cubes

1. In a blender, combine the coconut milk, spinach, banana, avocado, cucumber, mint, lemon juice, and honey. Blend until smooth.
2. Add the ice and blend until thick.

PER SERVING

Calories 482| Total fat 40g| Saturated fat 28g| Carbohydrates 37g| Fiber 9g| Protein 6g

Blueberry-Millet Breakfast Bake

Prep time: 10 minutes|Cooking time:55 minutes|Serves 8

- 2 cups millet, soaked in water overnight
- 2 cups fresh, or frozen, blueberries
- 1¾ cups unsweetened applesauce
- ⅓ cup coconut oil, melted
- 2 teaspoons grated fresh ginger
- 1½ teaspoons ground cinnamon

1. Preheat the oven to 350°F.
2. In a fine-mesh sieve, drain and rinse the millet for 1 to 2 minutes.
3. Transfer to a large bowl.
4. Gently fold in the blueberries, applesauce, coconut oil, ginger, and cinnamon.
5. Pour the mixture into a 9-by-9-inch casserole dish.
6. Cover with aluminum foil.
7. Place the dish in the preheated oven and bake for 40 minutes.
8. Remove the foil and bake for 10 to 15 minutes more, or until lightly crisp on top.

PER SERVING

Calories 323| Total Fat 13g| Total Carbohydrates 48g| Sugar 9g| Fiber 6g| Protein 6g| Sodium 4mg

Savory Quinoa Breakfast Stew

Prep time: 5 minutes|Cooking time:17 minutes|Serves 1

- ¼ cup quinoa
- ¾ cup water, plus additional as needed
- ½ small broccoli head, finely chopped
- 1 carrot, grated
- ¼ teaspoon salt
- 1 tablespoon chopped fresh dill

1. In a fine-mesh strainer, rinse the quinoa well.
2. In a small pot set over high heat, stir together the quinoa and water. Bring to a boil.
3. Reduce the heat to low. Cover and cook for 5 minutes.
4. Add the broccoli, carrot, and salt. Cook for 10 to 12 minutes more, or until the quinoa is fully cooked and tender.
5. If the stew gets too dry, add more water.
6. This should be on the liquid side as opposed to the drier consistency of a pilaf.
7. Fold in the dill and serve.

PER SERVING

Calories 220| Total Fat 3g| Total Carbohydrates 41g| Sugar 5g| Fiber 7g| Protein 10g| Sodium 667mg

"Choose Your Adventure" Chia Breakfast Pudding

Prep time: 5 minutes|Cooking time:0 minutes|Serves 4

- ¾ cup chia seeds
- ½ cup hemp seeds
- 2¼ cups coconut milk
- ½ cup dried cranberries
- ¼ cup maple syrup

1. In a medium bowl, stir together the chia seeds, hemp seeds, coconut milk, cranberries, and maple syrup, ensuring that the chia is completely mixed with the milk.
2. Cover the bowl and refrigerate overnight.
3. In the morning, stir and serve.

PER SERVING

Calories 483| Total Fat 41g| Total Carbohydrates 25g| Sugar 17g| Fiber 6g| Protein 9g| Sodium 22mg

Creamy Pistachio Smoothie

Prep time: 5 minutes|Cooking time:10 minutes|Serves 2

- 1 cup unsweetened almond milk
- 1 cup shredded kale
- 2 frozen bananas
- ½ cup shelled pistachios
- 2 tablespoons pure maple syrup
- 1 teaspoon pure vanilla extract

1. In a blender, combine the milk, kale, bananas, pistachios, maple syrup, and vanilla.
2. Blend until smooth and thick.

PER SERVING

Calories 275| Total fat 4g| Saturated fat 1g| Carbohydrates 48g| Fiber 5g| Protein 6g

Tropical Red Smoothie

Prep time: 5 minutes|Cooking time:10 minutes|Serves 2

- 1 cup coconut water
- ½ cup unsweetened pineapple juice
- 1 banana
- ½ cup fresh raspberries
- ½ cup unsweetened shredded coconut
- 3 ice cubes

1. In a blender, combine the coconut water, pineapple juice, banana, raspberries, and coconut. Blend until smooth.
2. Add the ice and blend until thick.

PER SERVING

Calories 209| Total fat 10g| Saturated fat 8g| Carbohydrates 31g| Fiber 7g| Protein 3g

Sweet Potato Pie Smoothie

Prep time: 5 minutes|Cooking time:10 minutes|Serves 2

- ½ cup unsweetened almond milk
- ½ cup freshly squeezed orange juice
- 1 cup cooked sweet potato
- 1 banana
- 2 tablespoons pumpkin seeds
- 1 tablespoon pure maple syrup
- ½ teaspoon pure vanilla extract
- ½ teaspoon ground cinnamon
- 3 ice cubes

1. In a blender, combine the almond milk, orange juice, sweet potato, banana, pumpkin seeds, maple syrup, vanilla, and cinnamon.
2. Blend until smooth.
3. Add the ice and blend until thick.

PER SERVING

Calories 235| Total fat 4g| Saturated fat 1g| Carbohydrates 43g| Fiber 6g| Protein 5g

Apple-Honey Smoothie

Prep time: 5 minutes|Cooking time:10 minutes|Serves 2

- 1 cup canned lite coconut milk
- 1 apple, cored and cut into chunks
- 1 banana
- ¼ cup almond butter
- 1 tablespoon raw honey
- ½ teaspoon ground cinnamon
- 4 ice cubes

1. In a blender, combine the coconut milk, apple, banana, almond butter, honey, and cinnamon. Blend until smooth.
2. Add the ice and blend until thick.

PER SERVING

Calories 434| Total fat 30g| Saturated fat 26g| Carbohydrates 46g| Fiber 8g| Protein 4g

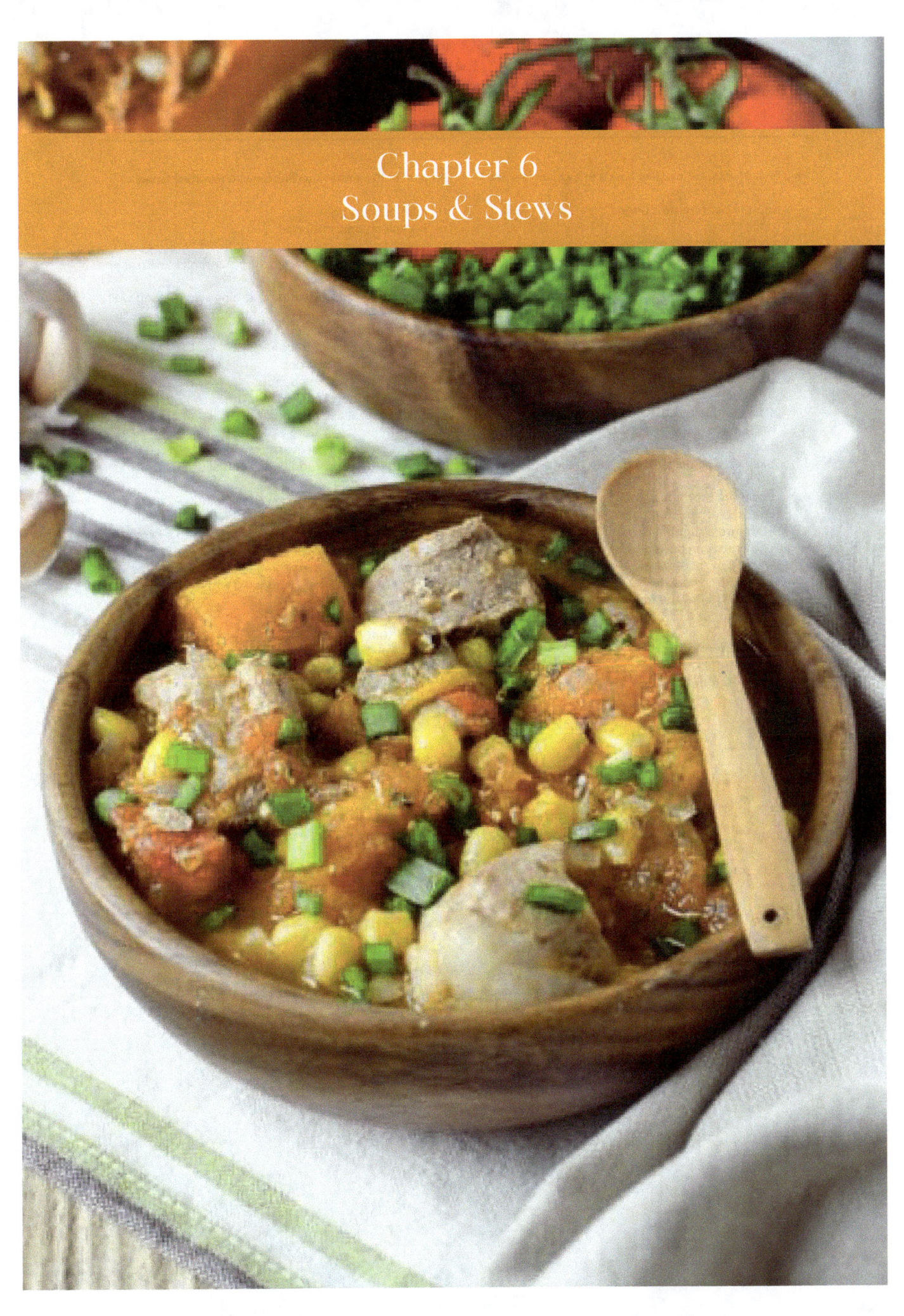

Chapter 6
Soups & Stews

Gut-Healing Bone Broth

Prep time: 15 minutes | Cooking time: 8 to 24 hours | Serves 4

- 2 pounds beef marrow bones
- 4 garlic cloves
- 3 medium carrots, chopped
- 2 celery stalks, chopped
- 1 medium onion, chopped
- 2 bay leaves
- 1 tablespoon apple cider vinegar
- Filtered water, to cover

1. In a 6-quart slow cooker, combine the bones, garlic, carrots, celery, onion, bay leaves, and vinegar.
2. Cover with filtered water. Set the cooker on low and simmer for at least 8 hours and up to 24 hours.
3. Skim off and discard any foam that forms on the surface.
4. Ladle the broth through a fine-mesh sieve or cheesecloth to strain out the solids.
5. Pour into airtight glass containers.
6. The broth can be kept refrigerated for up to 1 week; just reboil it before use. To freeze, allow the broth to completely cool and then fill jars up to 1 inch below the top to allow for expansion, and keep for 4 to 5 months.

PER SERVING

Calories 40| Total Fat 0g| Saturated Fat 0g| Cholesterol 0mg| Carbohydrates 5g| Fiber 0g| Protein 6g

Chicken Chili Blanco

Prep time: 10 minutes | Cooking time: 20 minutes | Serves 4

- 1 tablespoon ghee
- 2 small onions, chopped
- 6 garlic cloves, minced
- 2 (4-ounce) cans diced mild green chiles with their liquid
- 4 cups cooked white beans, drained and rinsed well
- 4 cups chicken broth or vegetable broth
- 4 teaspoons ground cumin
- 2 teaspoons dried oregano
- 1 teaspoon chili powder
- ¼ teaspoon cayenne pepper
- 4 cups shredded cooked chicken
- 2 scallions, sliced

1. In a large soup pot over medium heat, melt the ghee.
2. Add the onions and garlic, and sauté for 5 minutes.
3. Add the chiles, and cook for 2 minutes, stirring.
4. Stir in the beans, broth, cumin, oregano, chili powder, and cayenne pepper. Bring to a simmer.
5. Add the chicken, bring to a simmer, reduce the heat to medium-low, and cook for 10 minutes. Serve immediately, sprinkled with the scallions.

PER SERVING

Calories 304| Total Fat 4g| Saturated Fat 2g| Cholesterol 0mg| Carbohydrates 46g| Fiber 12g| Protein 21g

Mixed Berry Salad with Ginger
Prep time: 10 minutes|Cooking time:10 minutes|Serves 4

- 1 cup fresh blueberries
- 1 cup fresh raspberries
- 1 cup fresh strawberries
- 1 tablespoon grated fresh ginger
- zest of 1 orange
- juice of 1 orange

1. In a medium bowl, stir together the blueberries, raspberries, strawberries, ginger, orange zest, and orange juice to mix well.

PER SERVING

Calories 75| Total Fat <1g| Total Carbs 18g| Sugar 11g| Fiber 5g| Protein 1g| Sodium 1mg

Tomato and Basil Salad
Prep time: 10 minutes|Cooking time:10 minutes|Serves 4

- 4 large heirloom tomatoes, chopped
- ¼ cup fresh basil leaves, torn
- 2 garlic cloves, finely minced
- ¼ cup extra-virgin olive oil
- ½ teaspoon sea salt
- ¼ teaspoon freshly ground black pepper

1. In a medium bowl, gently mix together the tomatoes, basil, garlic, olive oil, salt, and pepper.

PER SERVING

Calories 140| Total Fat 14g| Total Carbs 4g| Sugar 3g| Fiber 1g| Protein 1g| Sodium 239mg

Pear-Walnut Salad
Prep time: 10 minutes|Cooking time:10 minutes|Serves 4

- 4 pears, peeled, cored, and chopped
- ¼ cup walnuts, chopped
- 2 tablespoons honey
- 2 tablespoons balsamic vinegar
- 2 tablespoons extra-virgin olive oil

1. In a medium bowl, combine the pears and walnuts.
2. In a small bowl, whisk the honey, balsamic vinegar, and olive oil.
3. Toss with the pears and walnuts.

PER SERVING

Calories 263| Total Fat 12g| Total Carbs 41g| Sugar 29g| Fiber 7g| Protein 3g| Sodium 3mg

Classic French Onion Soup
Prep time: 15 minutes|Cooking time:2 hour 30 minutes|Serves 4

- 2 tablespoons olive oil
- 3 pounds sweet onions, halved and cut into ⅛-inch-thick slices
- 2 teaspoons bottled minced garlic
- ½ cup dry sherry
- 8 cups Beef Bone Broth
- 1 tablespoon chopped fresh thyme
- Sea salt
- Freshly ground black pepper

1. Place a large stockpot over low heat and add the olive oil.
2. Add the onions and garlic. Cover the pot and cook for 30 minutes, letting the juices purge from the onions. Stir occasionally.
3. Remove the lid. Continue to sauté the onions and garlic, stirring occasionally, for about 1 hour, 30 minutes, or until they are a deep caramel color.
4. Add the sherry and deglaze the pan, scraping up any browned bits from the bottom.
5. Increase the heat to medium. Stir in the beef broth and thyme. Bring the soup to a boil. Reduce the heat to low and simmer for about 30 minutes, or until the onions are tender.
6. Season with sea salt and pepper.

PER SERVING

Calories 234| Total fat 9g| Saturated fat 2g| Carbohydrates 33g| Fiber 8g| Protein 9g

Slow-Cooker Vegan Split Pea Soup

Prep time: 10 minutes|Cooking time:4 to 8 hours|Serves 8

- 6½ cups water
- 2½ cups green or yellow split peas, rinsed well
- 2 small sweet potatoes, cut into ½-inch dice
- 1 tablespoon dried thyme
- 1½ teaspoons salt, plus additional as needed

1. In a slow cooker, combine the water, split peas, sweet potatoes, thyme, and salt.
2. Cover and cook on low for 8 hours, or on high for 4 hours.
3. Using an immersion blender or in a regular blender, blend half (or all) of the soup, working in batches as needed and taking care with the hot liquid.
4. Taste and adjust the seasoning, if necessary.

PER SERVING

Calories 51| Total Fat 0g| Total Carbohydrates 12g| Sugar 0g| Fiber 2g| Protein 1g| Sodium 448mg

Carrot Ginger Soup

Prep time: 10 minutes|Cooking time:30 minutes|Serves 6 to 8

- 1 large onion, peeled and roughly chopped
- 4½ cups plus 2 tablespoons water, divided
- 8 carrots, peeled and roughly chopped (see Tip)
- 1½-inch piece fresh ginger, sliced thin (see Tip)
- 1¼ teaspoons sea salt
- 2 cups unsweetened coconut milk

1. In a large pot set over medium heat, sauté the onion in 2 tablespoons of water for about 5 minutes, or until soft.
2. Add the carrots, the remaining 4½ cups of water, the ginger, and salt. Bring to a boil. Reduce the heat to low and cover the pot. Simmer for 20 minutes.
3. Stir in the coconut milk and let it heat for 4 to 5 minutes.
4. In a blender, blend the soup until creamy, working in batches if necessary and taking care with the hot liquid.

PER SERVING

Calories 228| Total Fat 19g| Total Carbohydrates 15g| Sugar 8g| Fiber 4g| Protein 3g| Sodium 554mg

Cream Of Broccoli Soup

Prep time: 12 minutes|Cooking time:25 minutes|Serves 6

- 1 onion, finely chopped
- 4 garlic cloves, finely chopped
- 5 cups plus 2 tablespoons water, divided
- 1½ teaspoons sea salt, plus additional as needed
- 4 broccoli heads with stalks, heads cut into florets and stalks roughly chopped
- 1 cup cashews, soaked in water for at least 4 hours

1. In a large pot set over medium heat, sauté the onion and garlic in 2 tablespoons of water for about 5 minutes, or until soft.
2. Add the remaining 5 cups of water, the salt, and the broccoli. Bring to a boil. Cover and reduce the heat to low. Simmer for 20 minutes.
3. Drain and rinse the cashews. Transfer them to a blender.
4. Add the soup to the blender. Blend until smooth, working in batches if necessary, and taking care with the hot liquid. Taste, and adjust the seasoning if necessary.

PER SERVING

Calories 224| Total Fat 11g| Total Carbohydrates 26g| Sugar 6g| Fiber 7g| Protein 11g| Sodium 85mg

Classic Butternut Squash Soup

Prep time: 20 minutes|Cooking time:30 minutes|Serves 6

- 1 onion, roughly chopped
- 4½ cups plus 2 tablespoons water, divided
- 1 large butternut squash, washed, peeled, ends trimmed, halved, seeded, and cut into ½-inch chunks
- 2 celery stalks, roughly chopped
- 3 carrots, peeled and roughly chopped
- 1 teaspoon sea salt, plus additional as needed

1. In a large pot set over medium heat, sauté the onion in 2 tablespoons of water for about 5 minutes, or until soft.
2. Add the squash, celery, carrot, and salt. Bring to a boil.
3. Reduce the heat to low, Cover and simmer for 25 minutes.
4. In a blender, purée the soup until smooth, working in batches if necessary and taking care with the hot liquid. Taste, and adjust the seasoning if necessary.

PER SERVING

Calories 104| Total Fat 0g| Total Carbohydrates 27g| Sugar 6g| Fiber 5g| Protein 2g| Sodium 417mg

Summer Vegetable Soup

Prep time: 20 minutes|Cooking time:35 minutes|Serves 4

- 1 tablespoon olive oil
- 2 stalks celery, chopped, or about ¾ to 1 cup precut packaged celery
- 1 sweet onion, chopped, or about 1 cup precut packaged onion
- 2 teaspoons bottled minced garlic
- 2 carrots, halved lengthwise and thinly sliced, or about 1 to 1½ cups precut packaged carrots
- 1 sweet potato, peeled and diced, or 1½ cups precut packaged sweet potatoes
- 8 cups low-sodium vegetable broth
- 2 cups (1-inch) green bean pieces
- 1 cup cauliflower florets
- 2 tablespoons chopped fresh basil
- Sea salt
- Freshly ground black pepper

1. In a large stockpot over medium-high heat, heat the olive oil.
2. Add the celery, onion, and garlic. Sauté for about 4 minutes, or until softened.
3. Add the carrots and sweet potato. Sauté for 3 minutes.
4. Stir in the vegetable broth. Bring the soup to a boil. Reduce the heat to low and simmer the soup for about 20 minutes, or until the vegetables are crisp-tender.
5. Stir in the green beans, cauliflower, and basil. Simmer for 5 minutes.
6. Season the soup with sea salt and pepper and serve.

PER SERVING

Calories 140| Total fat 4g| Saturated fat 1g| Carbohydrates 21g| Fiber 7g| Protein 4g

Chilled Coconut-Avocado Soup

Prep time: 15 minutes|Cooking time:1 hour|Serves 8

- 3 ripe avocados, peeled and pitted
- ¼ red onion, chopped, or about ¼ cup precut packaged onion
- 1 cup Herbed Chicken Bone Broth
- 1 tablespoon freshly squeezed lemon juice
- 1 garlic clove, crushed
- 1 teaspoon grated fresh ginger
- ½ teaspoon chopped fresh dill, plus fresh dill sprigs for garnish
- 2 cups canned full-fat coconut milk
- Sea salt
- Freshly ground black pepper
- Sliced radishes, for garnish

1. Coarsely chop three of the four avocado halves. Dice the remaining half and set it aside for garnish.
2. In a food processor, combine the chopped avocado, onion, chicken broth, lemon juice, garlic, ginger, and chopped dill. Purée until very smooth. Transfer the avocado soup to a lidded container.
3. Whisk in the coconut milk.
4. Season with sea salt and pepper. Chill the soup for at least 1 hour.
5. Garnish with the diced avocado, radishes, and dill sprigs just before serving.

PER SERVING

Calories 395| Total fat 39g| Saturated fat 21g| Carbohydrates 14g| Fiber 9g| Protein 4g

Chapter 7
Salads

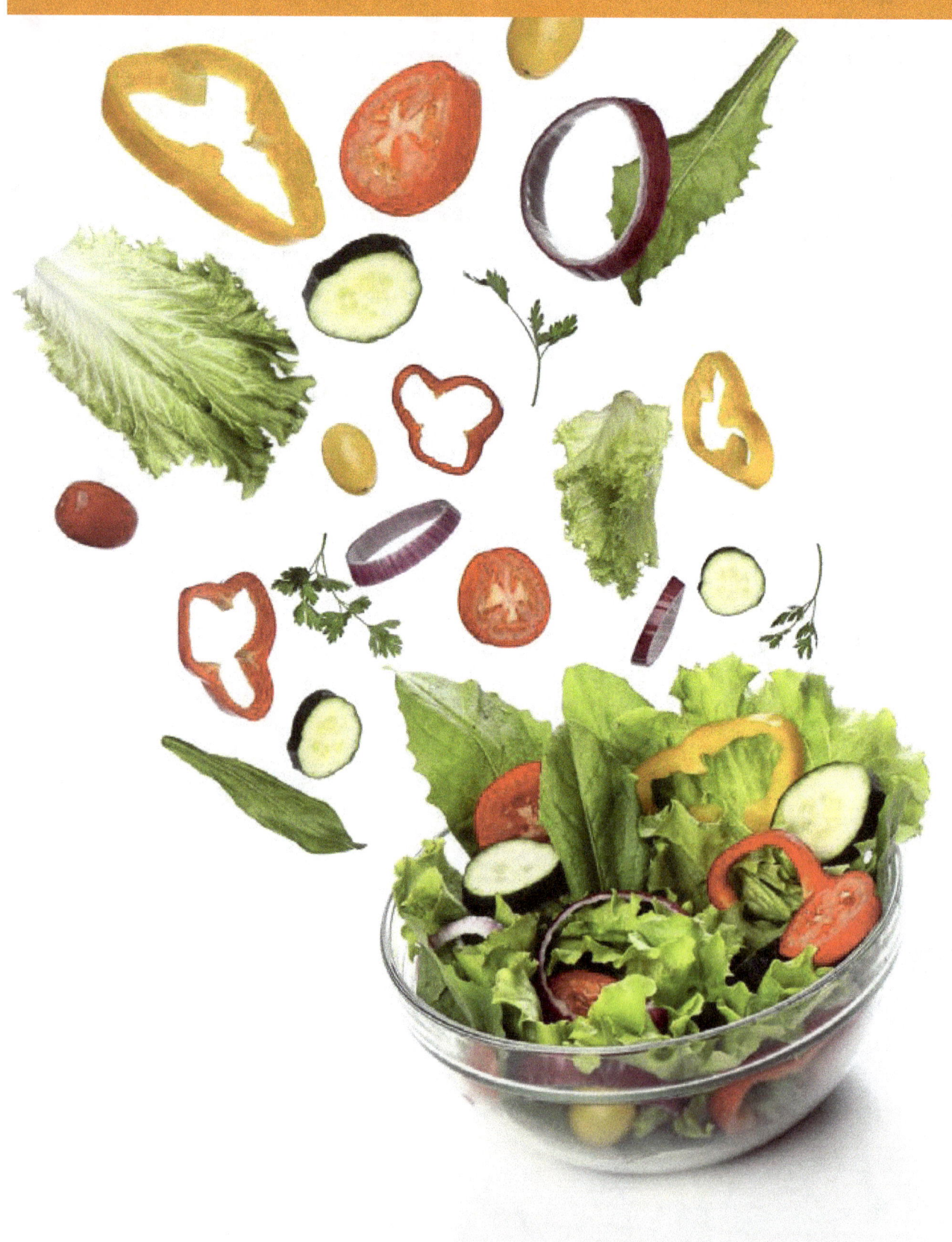

Massaged Kale Salad

Prep time: 15 minutes|Cooking time:10 minutes|Serves 4

- 2 bunches Lacinato kale, stemmed and torn into bite-size pieces
- 3 scallions, sliced
- 1 avocado, diced
- ¼ cup shelled sunflower seeds
- 2 tablespoons freshly squeezed lemon juice
- 3 tablespoons extra-virgin olive oil
- ½ teaspoon salt
- Freshly ground black pepper
- ¼ cup pomegranate seeds

1. In a large bowl, combine the kale, scallions, avocado, sunflower seeds, lemon juice, olive oil, and salt, and season with pepper.
2. With your hands, massage the salad ingredients for about 5 minutes until the kale begins to soften and the avocado is creamed into the other ingredients.
3. Mix the pomegranate seeds into the salad and serve immediately.

PER SERVING

Calories 249| Total Fat 21g| Saturated Fat 3g| Cholesterol 0mg| Carbohydrates 14g| Fiber 6g| Protein 6g

Shaved Brussels Sprout Salad

Prep time: 15 minutes|Cooking time:10 minutes|Serves 4

- 1 pound Brussels sprouts, trimmed and thinly sliced into ribbons from top to stem (discard the stems)
- 2 hard-boiled eggs, peeled and roughly chopped
- ¼ cup pine nuts
- 3 tablespoons freshly squeezed lemon juice
- 3 tablespoons extra-virgin olive oil
- 1 tablespoon minced shallot
- Pinch salt
- Freshly ground black pepper

1. In a large bowl, toss together the Brussels sprouts, eggs, pine nuts, lemon juice, olive oil, and shallot.
2. Sprinkle with the salt and season with pepper.

PER SERVING

Calories 213| Total Fat 17.3g| Saturated Fat 2.2g| Cholesterol 54.6mg| Carbohydrates 10.7g| Fiber 4.7g| Protein 7.1g

Spicy Broccoli Slaw

Prep time: 10 minutes|Cooking time:10 minutes|Serves 4

- 1 head broccoli, roughly chopped into bite-size pieces
- 2 scallions, sliced
- ¼ cup sliced almonds
- ¼ cup dried cranberries
- 2 tablespoons plain whole-milk yogurt
- 1 tablespoon Paleo mayonnaise
- 1 tablespoon freshly squeezed lemon juice
- 1 teaspoon raw honey
- ½ teaspoon ground cumin
- Dash hot sauce
- Freshly ground black pepper

1. In a large bowl, combine the broccoli, scallions, almonds, and cranberries.
2. In a small bowl, whisk the yogurt, mayonnaise, lemon juice, honey, cumin, hot sauce, and salt, and season with pepper.
3. Pour this dressing over the broccoli mixture and stir well to combine.

PER SERVING

Calories 110| Total Fat 7g| Saturated Fat 1g| Cholesterol 6mg| Carbohydrates 12g| Fiber 2g| Protein 2g

Rainbow Bean Salad

Prep time: 10 minutes|Cooking time:0 minutes|Serves 4

- For the dressing
- ½ cup extra-virgin olive oil
- 1 tablespoon freshly squeezed lime juice
- ½ teaspoon garlic powder
- ½ teaspoon chili powder
- ½ teaspoon salt
- ¼ teaspoon red pepper flakes
- For the salad
- 3 cups cooked wild rice
- 2 cups cooked black beans, drained and rinsed well
- 1 cup non-GMO organic sweet corn kernels
- 1 red bell pepper, diced
- 4 scallions, sliced
- ¼ cup chopped fresh cilantro

TO MAKE THE DRESSING

1. In a small bowl, whisk the olive oil, vinegar, lime juice, garlic powder, chili powder, salt, red pepper flakes, and black pepper.
2. Set aside.

TO MAKE THE SALAD

1. In a medium bowl, stir together the rice, beans, corn, red bell pepper, scallions, and cilantro.
2. Pour the dressing over the vegetables and toss to coat evenly. Serve chilled, if desired.

PER SERVING

Calories 423| Total Fat 24g| Saturated Fat 3g| Cholesterol 0mg| Carbohydrates 47g| Fiber 17g| Protein 13g

Green Pasta Salad

Prep time: 15 minutes|Cooking time:15 minutes|Serves 6-8

- 1 (12-ounce) package gluten-free penne or fusilli
- 1 bunch asparagus, sliced on the diagonal into 1-inch pieces
- 1 tablespoon extra-virgin olive oil
- 1 cup Tofu-Basil Sauce
- 2 cups arugula
- 2 scallions, sliced
- 1 teaspoon salt
- ¼ teaspoon freshly ground black pepper

1. Cook the pasta in a large pot of boiling water according to the package directions.
2. Add the asparagus to the pot for the last 2 minutes of cooking time. Drain the pasta and asparagus in a colander, then return them to the pot.
3. Add the olive oil and sauce and stir to combine.
4. Set aside to cool to room temperature.
5. Stir in the arugula, scallions, salt, and pepper and serve.

PER SERVING

Calories 450| Total Fat 15g| Total Carbohydrates 68g| Sugar 3g| Fiber 5g| Protein 13g| Sodium 290mg

Carrot And Raisin Salad

Prep time: 12 minutes|Cooking time:0 minutes|Serves 6

- 4 cups shredded carrots
- 1 cup raisins, chopped
- ¾ cup sunflower seeds
- ¼ cup maple syrup, plus additional as needed
- ¼ cup freshly squeezed lemon juice, plus additional as needed

1. In a large bowl, mix together the carrots, raisins, and sunflower seeds.
2. Stir in the maple syrup and lemon juice.
3. Taste, and add more lemon juice or maple syrup if necessary.

PER SERVING

Calories 173| Total Fat 3g| Total Carbohydrates 37g| Sugar 26g| Fiber 3g| Protein 3g| Sodium 57mg

Chilled Sweet Potato Salad

Prep time: 12 minutes|Cooking time:20 minutes|Serves 6

- 4 sweet potatoes, or yams, cut into ½-inch cubes
- 2 scallions, finely chopped
- ½ cup fresh dill, finely chopped
- ¼ cup extra-virgin olive oil
- 1½ teaspoons salt

1. Fill a large pot with 3 to 4 inches of water and insert a steamer basket. Bring the water to a boil over high heat.
2. Add the sweet potatoes to the steamer basket.
3. Depending on the size of your basket, you may need to do this in two batches.
4. Cover and steam for 8 to 10 minutes, or until the potatoes are firm and tender, but not mushy.
5. Drain, and rinse under cold water to stop the cooking process.
6. In a large bowl, gently combine the sweet potatoes, scallions, dill, olive oil, and salt.
7. Refrigerate until ready to serve.

PER SERVING

Calories 241| Total Fat 9g| Total Carbohydrates 40g| Sugar 1g| Fiber 6g| Protein 3g| Sodium 601mg

Quinoa Lentil Salad

Prep time: 20 minutes|Cooking time:45 minutes|Serves 6

- 1 cup green, brown, or French green lentils
- 4 cups water, divided
- 1 cup quinoa
- 1 broccoli head, finely chopped
- 4 carrots, grated
- ⅓ cup extra-virgin olive oil
- 1 teaspoon salt, plus additional as needed

1. In a fine-mesh strainer, rinse the lentils.
2. Transfer to a medium pot set over high heat and add 2 cups of water. Bring to a boil.
3. Simmer for 15 to 20 minutes, or until tender. Drain off any excess liquid.
4. In a fine-mesh strainer, rinse the quinoa.
5. Transfer to another medium pot set over high heat and add the remaining 2 cups of water.
6. Bring to a boil. Simmer for 15 minutes, or until all the liquid is absorbed.
7. Remove from the heat and let sit for 10 minutes. Fluff with a fork.
8. In a large bowl, combine the lentils, quinoa, broccoli, and carrots.
9. Stir in the olive oil and salt.
10. Taste and adjust the seasoning, if necessary.
11. Refrigerate for at least 1 hour before serving.

PER SERVING

Calories 369| Total Fat 16g| Total Carbohydrates 44g| Sugar 3g| Fiber 14g| Protein 14g| Sodium 434mg

Crispy Kale Salad

Prep time: 10 minutes|Cooking time:20 minutes|Serves 6

- 15 ounces kale, stemmed, thoroughly washed and dried, and chopped into bite-size pieces
- 3 tablespoons extra-virgin olive oil
- 2 tablespoons apple cider vinegar
- 1 teaspoon salt
- ½ teaspoon red pepper flakes
- ¼ teaspoon freshly ground black pepper
- 1 small leek, white and pale green parts, thoroughly washed (see Ingredient Tip)
- 2 small sweet potatoes, peeled
- 1 apple, peeled
- 1 tablespoon avocado oil
- ¼ cup pine nuts

1. Preheat the oven to 350°F.
2. Line a backing sheet with parchment paper.
3. In a large bowl, combine the kale, olive oil, vinegar, salt, and red pepper flakes, and season with black pepper. With your hands, knead the oil and spices into the kale for 1 minute. Transfer three-fourths of the kale to the prepared pan and spread it evenly. Bake for 20 minutes, tossing halfway through. Set aside the bowl with the rest of the kale.
4. While the kale cooks, chop the leek, sweet potatoes, and apple into bite-size pieces. Add with the avocado oil to a large skillet over medium heat, and sauté for about 10 minutes, until the sweet potatoes soften.
5. Remove the crispy kale from the oven and add it to the reserved uncooked kale.
6. Top with the sweet potato mixture and the pine nuts, and mix well.
7. Serve warm.

PER SERVING

Calories 213| Total Fat 14g| Saturated Fat 2g| Cholesterol 0mg| Carbohydrates 22g| Fiber 5g| Protein 5g

Stone Fruit Salad

Prep time: 15 minutes|Cooking time:10 minutes|Serves 6

- 4 cups mixed chopped greens
- 1 cup sliced fresh peaches
- 1 cup fresh cherries, pitted and halved
- 1 cup sliced fresh nectarines
- ½ cup pecans, chopped
- ¼ cup thinly sliced red onion
- ¼ cup fresh basil leaves
- ⅓ cup extra-virgin olive oil
- ¼ cup balsamic vinegar
- 1 tablespoon freshly squeezed lemon juice
- ½ tablespoon raw honey
- Dash salt
- Freshly ground black pepper

1. In a large bowl, gently combine the greens, peaches, cherries, nectarines, pecans, red onion, and basil.
2. In a small bowl, add the olive oil, vinegar, lemon juice, honey, and salt, season with pepper, and whisk to combine.
3. Pour the dressing over the salad and gently toss to combine. Serve immediately.

PER SERVING

Calories 235| Total Fat 19g| Saturated Fat 2g| Cholesterol 0mg| Carbohydrates 16g| Fiber 3g| Protein 2g

Warm Fig & Sweet Potato Salad

Prep time: 10 minutes|Cooking time:20 minutes|Serves 6

- 4 sweet potatoes, cubed
- 6 tablespoons extra-virgin olive oil, divided
- 1 teaspoon salt
- 6 ripe fresh figs, quartered
- 2 tablespoons balsamic vinegar
- 1 teaspoon Dijon mustard
- 1 teaspoon raw honey
- 3 scallions, sliced
- 1 red chile pepper, such as serrano, seeded and thinly sliced
- Freshly ground black pepper
- Crumbled goat cheese, for garnishing (optional)

1. Preheat the oven to 475°F.
2. Line a baking sheet with aluminum foil.
3. In a large bowl, toss the sweet potato cubes in 3 tablespoons of olive oil and the salt.
4. Spread on the prepared pan and roast for 20 minutes. Halfway through, flip the potatoes and add the figs.
5. Meanwhile, in a small bowl, whisk 2 tablespoons of olive oil with the vinegar, mustard, and honey. Set the dressing aside.
6. In a small skillet over medium heat, sauté the scallions and red chile in the remaining 1 tablespoon of olive oil for 2 minutes.
7. In a large bowl, combine the roasted sweet potatoes and figs with the scallions and the red chile. Pour the dressing over and gently stir to combine.
8. Season with pepper and sprinkle with goat cheese (if using). Serve warm.

PER SERVING

Calories 253| Total Fat 14g| Saturated Fat 2g| Cholesterol 0mg| Carbohydrates 32g| Fiber 5g| Protein 2g

Chapter 8
Eggs

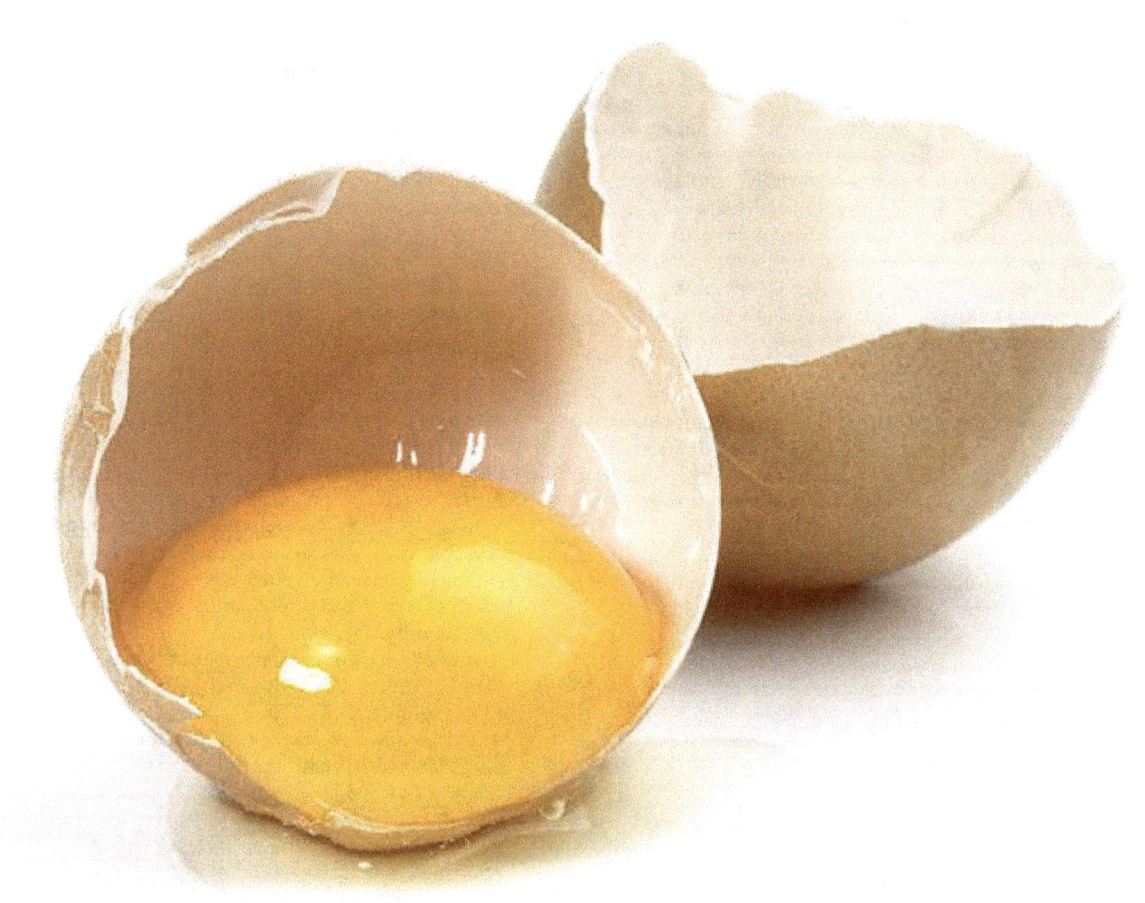

kailua breakfast bowl

Prep time: 5 minutes|Cooking time:7 minutes|Serves 1

- 1 large egg
- 1 tablespoon avocado oil
- 5 or 6 leaves curly or dinosaur kale, chopped (about 1 cup)
- ¼ teaspoon fine Himalayan salt
- 2 tablespoons Coconut Yogurt
- ¼ cup Carne Molida
- 2 tablespoons Pickled Red Onions

1. Bring a small pot of water to a rapid boil over high heat.
2. In the meantime, heat a large skillet over medium heat.
3. When the water begins to boil, gently add the egg and set a timer for 6 minutes.
4. While the egg cooks, pour the avocado oil into the skillet and add the kale.
5. Sprinkle with the salt. Sauté, stirring often, until the kale wilts and begins to brown, about 6 minutes.
6. Remove from the heat and transfer the kale to a serving plate.
7. After 6 minutes, remove the pot with the egg from the heat and drain the water, leaving the egg in the pot.
8. Fill the pot with cool water and ice, enough to cover the egg.
9. Let the egg sit in the ice bath for 2 minutes while you prepare the rest of the dish.
10. Smear the yogurt on the plate across from the kale.
11. Spoon the carne molida between the kale and the yogurt and top with the pickled onions.
12. Tap the egg on the counter to crack the shell and then submerge it under the water to peel it.
13. Place the egg on the yogurt and use a paring knife to make a vertical slit in it, letting the yolk spill out over the yogurt.
14. Serve right away and dig in! The best way to store this dish is by storing the different components in separate airtight containers in the fridge for up to 5 days.

PER SERVING

Calories 478 | Fat 31.3g | Total Carbohydrate 12.5g | Dietary Fiber 2.3g | Protein 33.6g

Mini Quiche Muffins

Prep time: 15 minutes|Cooking time:35 minutes|Serves 12

- For the filling:
- 4 slices bacon, diced
- 2 cups rainbow slaw (see Note)
- 1 teaspoon fine Himalayan salt, divided
- 5 large eggs
- ½ teaspoon ground black pepper
- ½ teaspoon dried Italian herb blend
- ½ cup full-fat coconut milk
- ¼ cup nutritional yeast
- For the crust:
- ¼ cup coconut flour
- 4 to 5 tablespoons flaxseed meal
- ¼ cup lard, unsalted butter, or ghee, softened
- 1 to 3 tablespoons ice-cold water

1. Preheat the oven to 400°F.
2. Line a standard-size 12-cup muffin tin with baking cups and lightly grease them with coconut oil or avocado oil.
3. In a large skillet, cook the bacon over medium-high heat until crispy, stirring occasionally.
4. Remove the bacon from the skillet and set it on a plate to cool, leaving the fat in the skillet.
5. Add the rainbow slaw and ½ teaspoon of the salt to the skillet. Cover and cook for about 10 minutes, stirring occasionally.
6. While the slaw cooks, make the crust: Mix together the coconut flour and flaxseed meal in a small bowl.
7. Add the lard and use your fingertips to break it up until a crumbly dough forms.
8. Add the water a tablespoon at a time, until the dough comes together and you can form it into a large ball.
9. Cover the bowl and place it in the fridge.
10. The slaw should be done by now.
11. Remove the skillet from the heat and transfer the slaw to the plate with the bacon to cool.
12. In a large bowl, whisk together the eggs, the remaining ½ teaspoon of salt, the seasonings, and the coconut milk.
13. Add the nutritional yeast and whisk until well combined but not too frothy.
14. Grab the dough from the fridge.
15. Break off ½-inch pieces and press them down into the bottoms of the baking cups, creating little crusts.
16. Par-bake the crusts for 5 minutes.
17. While the crusts par-bake, mix the cooled slaw and bacon into the egg mixture.
18. Remove the crusts from the oven and ladle the egg-and-slaw mixture into the muffin cups, filling them three-quarters full.
19. Bake for 15 minutes, or until the centers are set and the muffins are fluffy and golden.
20. Let cool for 5 minutes before serving.
21. Store in an airtight container in the fridge for up to 1 week.
22. To reheat, toast in a preheated 350°F oven for 8 minutes or microwave on high for 1 minute.

PER SERVING

Calories 155 | Fat 12.5g | Total Carbohydrate 4.6g | Dietary Fiber 2.3g | Protein 6.6g

Greek-Style Egg Muffins with Broccoli

Prep time: 5 minutes|Cooking time:30 minutes|Serves 4

- 2 tbsp olive oil
- 2 tbsp Greek-style yogurt
- 1 onion, chopped
- 1 cup diced broccoli florets
- 8 eggs, beaten
- 1 tsp garlic powder
- Sea salt and pepper to taste

1. Preheat your oven to 350°F.
2. Grease a muffin tin with cooking spray.
3. Warm the oil in a skillet over medium heat, place the onion and broccoli, and cook for 3 minutes.
4. Divide the veggies between 4 muffin cups.
5. Beat the eggs, yogurt, garlic powder, salt, and pepper in a bowl and pour it over the veggies.
6. Bake for 15-17 minutes until the eggs are set.
7. Serve and enjoy!

PER SERVING

Cal 210| Fat 17| Carbs 6g| Protein 1g

Avocado & Egg Salad Lettuce Cups

Prep time: 5 minutes|Cooking time:10 minutes|Serves 4

- 1 avocado, stoned and diced
- 2 tbsp cilantro, chopped
- 8 hard-boiled eggs, chopped
- ¼ cup paleo mayonnaise
- 1 tsp Dijon mustard
- Sea salt and pepper to taste
- 4 large lettuce leaves

1. Mix the avocado, eggs, cilantro, mayonnaise, mustard, salt, and pepper in a bowl until well combined.
2. Spoon the salad into each lettuce leaf and serve well-chilled.

PER SERVING

Cal 200| Fat 15| Carbs 7g| Protein 1g

Pressure Cooked Deviled Eggs

Prep time: 5 minutes|Cooking time:20 minutes|Serves 4

- 4 eggs
- 1 tsp paprika
- 1 tbsp paleo mayonnaise
- 1 tsp Dijon mustard

1. Place the eggs and 1 cup of water in your Instant Pot.
2. Close the lid and cook for 5 minutes on "Manual".
3. Let the pressure release naturally.
4. Place the eggs in an ice bath and let cool for 5 minutes.
5. Peel and cut them in half.
6. Whisk together the remaining ingredients.
7. Top the egg halves with the mixture and enjoy!

PER SERVING

Cal 100| Fat 8g| Carbs 0.7g| Protein 6g

Crispy Eggs + Cabbage

Prep time: 5 minutes|Cooking time:10 minutes|Serves 1

- 1 tablespoon coconut oil or avocado oil
- ½ medium head cabbage, sliced (about 2 cups)
- 2 slices prosciutto, ham, or bacon
- 2 large eggs
- ½ teaspoon fine Himalayan salt

1. Heat an 8-inch skillet or griddle over medium heat.
2. When it's hot, melt the oil in the skillet, swirling it around to grease the entire surface.
3. Add the cabbage, distributing it evenly over the whole skillet in one even layer.
4. Let it cook undisturbed for about 5 minutes, until the bottom of the cabbage browns.
5. Move the cabbage to one side of the skillet, forming a little mound.
6. Put the prosciutto slices on the other side of the skillet and cook for 2 to 3 minutes, until crispy, flipping once.
7. Then push the prosciutto to the side, snuggled up against the cabbage.
8. Crack the eggs into the remaining space in the skillet and sprinkle everything with the salt.
9. Let the eggs cook for 2 to 3 minutes, until the whites are no longer translucent and the edges are crispy.
10. If the eggs look done except for little pools of raw white near the yolk, use a spatula to gently distribute the loose egg white over the cooked egg parts until they too are cooked.
11. Serve right away.
12. You can even eat it right out of the skillet! If you have leftovers, store them covered in the fridge for up to 3 days.

PER SERVING

Calories 437 | Fat 33.6g | Total Carbohydrate 8.7g | Dietary Fiber 3.5g | Protein 30.4g

Broccoli Egg Cups

Prep time: 5 minutes|Cooking time:30 minutes|Serves 4

- 1 shallot, chopped
- 5 oz chopped broccoli florets
- 2 tbsp extra-virgin olive oil
- 8 eggs, beaten
- 1 tsp garlic powder
- Sea salt and pepper to taste

1. Preheat your oven to 350°F.
2. Spray a muffin tin with nonstick cooking spray.
3. Warm the olive oil in a skillet over medium heat.
4. Add the shallot and broccoli. Cook for 3 minutes.
5. Spoon the vegetables evenly into 4 muffin cups. In a medium bowl, beat the eggs, garlic powder, salt, and pepper.
6. Pour them over the vegetables in the muffin cups.
7. Bake for 15-17 minutes until the eggs set.

PER SERVING

Cal 205| Fat 15g| Carbs 5g| Protein 11g

Korean Style Lentils

Prep time: 5 minutes|Cooking time:30 minutes|Serves 4

- 2 spring onions, diced
- 2 garlic cloves, minced
- 2 cups vegetable broth
- 1 cup lentils
- 1 tbsp avocado oil
- 3 tbsp coconut aminos
- 2 tbsp coconut sugar
- 1 tbsp rice vinegar
- 1 tsp extra-virgin olive oil
- ½ tsp ground ginger
- ¼ tsp red pepper flakes
- 1 tbsp sesame seeds
- 2 scallions, sliced

1. Warm the avocado oil in a pot over medium heat.
2. Add the spring onions and garlic.
3. Sauté for 5 minutes, or until the onion is translucent.
4. Stir in the broth, lentils, coconut aminos, coconut sugar, vinegar, olive oil, ginger, and red pepper flakes.
5. Increase the heat to medium and bring to a simmer.
6. Reduce the heat to low, cover, and cook for 15 minutes, or until the lentils are cooked.
7. Garnish with sesame seeds and scallions. Serve and enjoy!

PER SERVING

Cal 280| Fat 6g| Carbs 45g| Protein 13g

Vegetarian Sloppy Joes

Prep time: 5 minutes|Cooking time:30 minutes|Serves 4

- 1 shallot, chopped
- 1 celery stalk, chopped
- 1 carrot, minced
- 2 garlic cloves, minced
- 1 lb cooked lentils
- ½ red bell pepper, chopped
- 2 tbsp avocado oil, divided
- 7 tbsp tomato paste
- 2 tbsp apple cider vinegar
- 1 tbsp pure maple syrup
- 1 tsp Dijon mustard
- 1 tsp chili powder
- ½ tsp dried oregano

1. Warm the avocado oil in a pan over medium heat.
2. Add the shallot, celery, carrot, and garlic, and sauté for about 3 minutes, or until the onion is translucent.
3. Add the lentils and the remaining avocado oil, and sauté for about 5 minutes.
4. Add the red bell pepper, and sauté for 2 minutes.
5. Stir in the tomato paste, vinegar, maple syrup, mustard, chili powder, and oregano.
6. Reduce the heat to medium-low and cook for about 10 minutes, stirring occasionally.
7. Serve over rice if desired.

PER SERVING

Cal 275| Fat 7g| Carbs 30g| Protein 13g

Eggs Benny

Prep time: 110 minutes|Cooking time:15 minutes|Serves 4

- 8 slices bacon
- 12 spears asparagus, trimmed
- 4 cups water
- 1 tablespoon white vinegar
- 4 large eggs
- 4 Savory Flax Waffles, for serving
- ¼ to ½ cup Hollandaise, for serving

1. Place the bacon slices on a sheet pan, spaced about 1 inch apart.
2. Distribute the asparagus around the bacon.
3. Place the sheet pan in the oven and set it to 400°F.
4. Cook until the oven comes to temperature, then for 10 to 15 more minutes.
5. Once the asparagus tips are lightly browned and the bacon is toasty on the edges, turn off the oven and crack the door a bit so everything stays warm. I like to put my waffles in there, too.
6. Begin poaching the eggs: Line a plate with paper towels. Heat the water in a small saucepan over medium heat.
7. Add the vinegar and bring to a steady simmer. Crack each of the eggs into its own small ramekin.
8. With a slotted spoon, stir the water in the saucepan to create a whirlpool, then slowly add an egg to the center of the whirlpool.
9. Gently stir the water around the edge of the pot for another 10 seconds, until the swirling motion of the water wraps the egg white around the yolk to create a neat poached egg.
10. Cook undisturbed for 3 minutes, until the white is opaque and the egg looks like a teardrop or a little ghost in the water.
11. Remove the egg from the water with a slotted spoon and place on the lined plate. Repeat with the remaining eggs.
12. Assemble the eggs bennys like so: a waffle on the bottom, a layer of asparagus, 2 slices of bacon, a poached egg, and then 1 to 2 tablespoons of hollandaise.
13. I don't recommend saving leftover poached eggs, as reheating them will cause them to overcook.
14. However, you can store the rest of the meal by packing each component separately in an airtight container.
15. They will keep in the fridge for up to 5 days.

PER SERVING

(without the hollandaise): Calories 410 | Fat 30.1g | Total Carbohydrate 11.7g | Dietary Fiber 9.7g | Protein 23.3g
Per 2 Tablespoons of hollandaise: Calories 112 | Fat 11.8g | Total Carbohydrate 0.7g | Dietary Fiber 0g | Protein 0.5g

Baked Scotch Eggs

Prep time: 10 minutes|Cooking time:35 minutes|Serves 8

- 6 cups water
- 8 large eggs
- 1 recipe Pork Sausage, uncooked
- 2 tablespoons avocado oil
- 2 tablespoons shelled hemp seeds (aka hemp hearts) (optional)
- 1 teaspoon fine Himalayan salt

1. Preheat the oven to 400°F.
2. Bring the water to a rapid boil in a large pot.
3. Gently place the eggs in the water and cook for 8 minutes.
4. Meanwhile, form the sausage mix into eight ¼-inch-thick, 4-inch-diameter patties.
5. Place them on a sheet of parchment paper or a cutting board and set aside.
6. When the eggs are done, drain the hot water from the pot, leaving the eggs in it, then fill the pot with cold water and ice.
7. Let the eggs chill in the ice bath for 2 minutes, then immediately peel them under the cold water.
8. Wrap the eggs: Place a pork patty in one hand. Using your other hand, place an egg in the center of the patty.
9. Close your hand holding the pork around the egg and use your other hand to pinch the sausage closed.
10. Gently shape the Scotch egg with both hands until it's smooth and even. Place the egg on a sheet pan, seam side down.
11. Repeat with the remaining eggs and pork patties.
12. Brush or spray the eggs with the oil. Sprinkle with the hemp seeds (if using) and salt. Bake for 25 minutes.
13. Remove from the oven and dig in! Or you can let the eggs cool and store in an airtight container in the refrigerator for up to 5 days.
14. I eat the leftovers cold, with a smear of Homemade Mayo on top.

PER SERVING

Calories 260 | Fat 20.2g | Total Carbohydrate 1.4g | Dietary Fiber 1.9g | Protein 17.1g

Egg Tart

Prep time: 20 minutes|Cooking time:20 minutes|Serves 4

- 1 cup Cheesy Yellow Sauce or Cauliflower Alfredo
- 1 baked Pie Crust
- 4 large eggs
- ¼ teaspoon fine Himalayan salt
- ¼ teaspoon ground black pepper
- 4 slices prosciutto di Parma

1. Spread the sauce evenly on the bottom of the baked pie crust.
2. Crack the eggs over the sauce and sprinkle with the salt and pepper.
3. Distribute the prosciutto slices around the eggs.
4. Wrap the edges of the crust in aluminum foil so they do not burn.
5. Bake for 20 minutes, or until the egg whites are completely set.
6. You can test this by gently shaking the pie to watch for a jiggle—when it doesn't move, it's done.
7. Remove from the oven and serve hot, or let cool and store in the refrigerator, covered, for up to 3 days.
8. To reheat, cut into four large slices, cover each slice with foil, and bake in a preheated 300°F oven for 10 minutes.

PER SERVING

Calories 471 | Fat 40.6g | Total Carbohydrate 9.2g | Dietary Fiber 6.3g | Protein 19.1g

Egg Roll-Ups

Prep time: 10 minutes|Cooking time:30 minutes|Serves 6

- 4 slices bacon
- 8 large eggs
- ¼ cup full-fat coconut milk
- ½ teaspoon fine Himalayan salt
- ½ teaspoon ground black pepper
- aby spinach
- 3 tablespoons Pistou

1. Lay the bacon slices flat on a 13 by 18-inch sheet pan, put it in the oven on the middle rack, and set the oven to 375°F.
2. Cook the bacon until the oven comes to temperature and then for up to 10 minutes more.
3. When it's crispy, remove it from the oven. Use a spatula to scrape it off the pan and set aside.
4. Drain some of the bacon grease off (into a receptacle to save it, of course). Line the greasy sheet pan with parchment paper.
5. Place the eggs, coconut milk, salt, and pepper in a blender. Blend on high for 45 seconds.
6. Pour the egg mixture into the prepared sheet pan.
7. Distribute the baby spinach evenly over the egg mixture.
8. Carefully place the sheet pan in the oven, using smooth and slow movements.

9. Bake for 10 minutes, or until the edges of the omelet begin to lift from the pan and the center is set.
10. Starting from the left side, roll the omelet until you have what looks like a giant egg roll.
11. Cut the roll into six pieces, serve, and enjoy! Store leftovers in an airtight container in the refrigerator for up to 5 days.
12. Enjoy them cold or gently reheat in the microwave on high for 30 seconds or in a 300°F oven for 5 minutes.

PER SERVING

Calories 432 | Fat 35.1g | Total Carbohydrate 4.2g | Dietary Fiber 1.6g | Protein 26g

Persian Herb Frittata

Prep time: 10 minutes|Cooking time:20 minutes|Serves 4

- 4 tablespoons avocado oil or olive oil, divided
- 1 large onion, diced
- 2 cloves garlic, minced
- 1 green onion, white part only, minced
- 6 large eggs
- 1 teaspoon baking powder (see Note)
- 1 teaspoon dried dill weed
- 1 teaspoon turmeric powder
- ½ teaspoon fine Himalayan salt
- ½ teaspoon ginger powder
- 1 cup minced fresh cilantro
- 1 cup minced fresh parsley
- ½ cup minced fresh basil

1. Heat an 8-inch skillet over medium or medium-low heat. If your stove runs hot, adjust the temperature; you don't want the bottom of the frittata to burn.
2. Remove the onion mix from the skillet and set aside to cool.
3. Put the skillet back on the stove over medium heat.
4. Cover with a tight-fitting lid.
5. Cook for 7 minutes, or until the edges of the frittata begin to separate from the skillet and the frittata is almost set but still wet in the center.
6. Then remove the lid and place the skillet under the broiler for 1 to 2 minutes.
7. Watch it carefully; you only need to broil it until the center is just set.
8. Remove the frittata from the oven.
9. Run a spatula around the edge of the frittata and carefully shake it out of the skillet and onto a cutting board.
10. Cut into four pieces, serve, and share.
11. Once the frittata has cooled to room temperature, you can store it in an airtight container in the refrigerator for up to 5 days.
12. Enjoy the leftovers cold or gently warmed up in a 300°F oven for 5 minutes.

PER SERVING

Calories 265 | Fat 22g | Total Carbohydrate 8g | Dietary Fiber 2g | Protein 11g

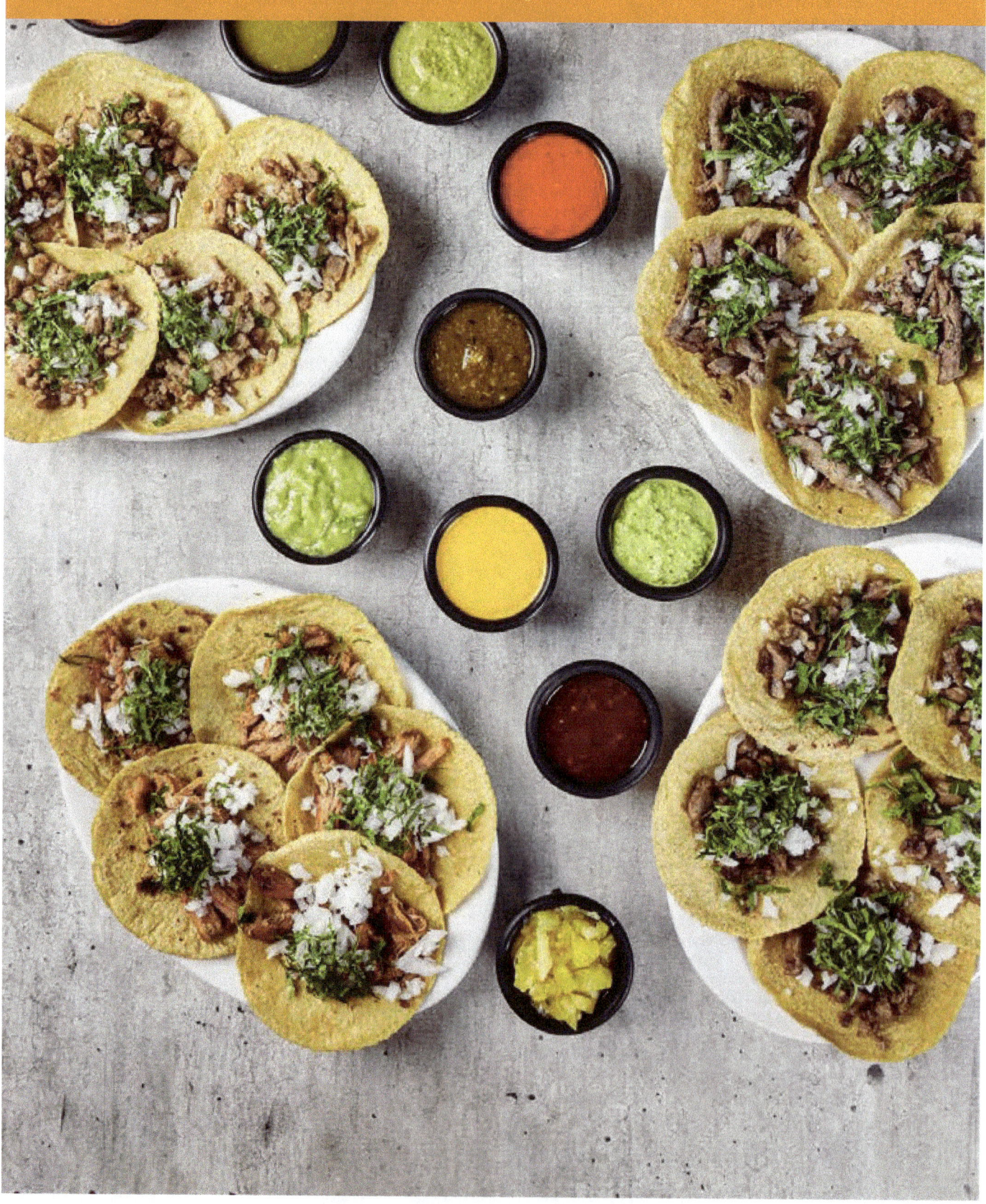

Chapter 9
Vegan & Vegetarian

Mixed Vegetable Stir-Fry

Prep time: 30 minutes|Cooking time:11 minutes|Serves 4

- ¼ cup low-sodium vegetable broth
- 1 tablespoon coconut aminos
- 2 teaspoons raw honey
- 1 teaspoon grated fresh ginger
- 1 teaspoon bottled minced garlic
- 1 teaspoon arrowroot powder
- 1½ teaspoons sesame oil
- 1 cup sliced mushrooms
- 2 carrots, thinly sliced, or about 1 to 1½ cups precut packaged carrots
- 1 celery stalk, thinly sliced on an angle, or ½ cup precut packaged celery
- 2 cups broccoli florets
- 1 cup cauliflower florets
- 1 cup snow peas, halved
- 1 cup bean sprouts
- ¼ cup chopped cashews
- 1 scallion, white and green parts, chopped

1. In a small bowl, whisk the vegetable broth, coconut aminos, honey, ginger, garlic, and arrowroot powder until well combined. Set it aside.
2. In a large skillet or wok over medium-high heat, heat the sesame oil.
3. Add the mushrooms, carrots, and celery. Sauté for 4 minutes.
4. Stir in the broccoli, cauliflower, and snow peas. Sauté for about 4 minutes until crisp-tender.
5. Add the bean sprouts and sauté for 1 minute.
6. Move the vegetables to one side of the skillet and add the sauce. Cook for about 2 minutes, stirring until the sauce has thickened. Stir the vegetables into the sauce, stirring to coat.
7. Serve topped with the cashews and scallion.

PER SERVING

Calories 154| Total fat 6g| Saturated fat 1g| Carbohydrates 21g| Fiber 4g| Protein 7g

Jam-Packed Peppers

Prep time: 15 minutes|Cooking time:4 to 5 hours|Serves 4

- 1 tablespoon avocado oil
- 4 bell peppers, any color, washed, tops cut off, and seeded
- ½ cup water
- 2 cups Spanish Rice
- 1 (15-ounce) can black beans, rinsed and drained well

1. Coat the bottom of the slow cooker with the avocado oil.
2. Place the peppers, upright, in the cooker.
3. Add the water to the bottom of the slow cooker, around the outside of the peppers.
4. In a large bowl, stir together the rice and black beans.
5. Stuff each pepper with one-quarter of the mixture.

6. Cover the cooker and set to low.
7. Cook for 4 to 5 hours and serve.

PER SERVING

Calories 340| Total Fat 9g| Total Carbs 58g| Sugar 3g| Fiber 7g| Protein 9g| Sodium 687mg

Sesame-Quinoa Cups

Prep time: 30 minutes|Cooking time:10 minutes|Serves 4

- For the dressing
- ¼ cup olive oil
- 2 tablespoons rice vinegar
- 1 tablespoon raw honey
- ½ teaspoon grated fresh ginger
- ½ teaspoon ground cumin
- Sea salt
- For the cups
- 1 cup cooked quinoa
- 1 cup shredded carrot
- 1 apple, cored and chopped
- 1 scallion, white and green parts, chopped
- ½ cup pumpkin seeds
- ¼ cup dried cranberries
- 1 tablespoon freshly squeezed lemon juice
- 1 large radicchio head, core removed, separated into 8 large leaves
- 1 tablespoon sesame seeds

TO MAKE THE DRESSING

1. In a small bowl, whisk the olive oil, rice vinegar, honey, ginger, and cumin. Season with sea salt and set it aside.

TO MAKE THE CUPS

1. In a large bowl, stir together the quinoa, carrot, apple, scallion, pumpkin seeds, cranberries, and lemon juice until well mixed.
2. Add the dressing and toss to mix well.
3. Spoon the rice mixture into the radicchio leaves, and serve topped with the sesame seeds.

PER SERVING

Calories 365| Total fat 23g| Saturated fat 4g| Carbohydrates 34g| Fiber 5g| Protein 8g

Indian-Spiced Cauliflower
Prep time: 15 minutes|Cooking time:3 to 4 hours|Serves 4 to 6

- 1 large head cauliflower, leaves and large stem removed
- ½ medium onion, diced
- 2 tablespoons extra-virgin olive oil
- ½ teaspoon sea salt
- ½ teaspoon garlic powder
- ½ teaspoon ground ginger
- ½ teaspoon curry powder
- ¼ teaspoon ground turmeric
- ¼ teaspoon ground cumin
- ⅛ teaspoon cayenne pepper

1. Chop the cauliflower into florets, and place them in the slow cooker with the onion.
2. In a small bowl, combine the olive oil, salt, garlic powder, ginger, curry powder, turmeric, cumin, and cayenne. Whisk into a paste. Using a pastry brush or a spoon, spread the spice paste onto the cauliflower florets.
3. Cover the cooker and set to low. Cook for 3 to 4 hours and serve.

PER SERVING

Calories 121| Total Fat 7g| Total Carbs 13g| Sugar 5g| Fiber 6g| Protein 4g| Sodium 354mg

Maple-Dijon Brussels Sprouts
Prep time: 15 minutes|Cooking time:3 to 4 hours|Serves 4 to 6

- 1 pound Brussels sprouts, ends trimmed
- 2 tablespoons maple syrup
- 1 tablespoon Dijon mustard
- ½ teaspoon garlic powder
- ½ teaspoon sea salt
- ¼ cup water

1. In your slow cooker, combine the Brussels sprouts, maple syrup, mustard, garlic powder, salt, and water. Toss together to distribute evenly.
2. Cover the cooker and set to low. Cook for 3 to 4 hours and serve.

PER SERVING

Calories 80| Total Fat 0g| Total Carbs 17g| Sugar 9g| Fiber 4g| Protein 4g| Sodium 410mg

Balsamic Beets
Prep time: 15 minutes|Cooking time:6 to 8 hours|Serves 6 to 8

- 4 to 6 medium beets (they need to fit snugly in the bottom of your slow cooker), chopped (see Tip)
- ½ cup balsamic vinegar
- 1 cup apple juice
- ½ teaspoon garlic powder
- ½ teaspoon dried rosemary
- Freshly ground black pepper

1. In your slow cooker, combine the beets, vinegar, apple juice, garlic powder, and rosemary, and season with pepper.
2. Cover the cooker and set to low. Cook for 6 to 8 hours and serve.

PER SERVING

Calories 96| Total Fat 0g| Total Carbs 21g| Sugar 13g| Fiber 1g| Protein 0g| Sodium 87mg

Thai Cabbage Bowl
Prep time: 20 minutes|Cooking time:15 minutes|Serves 4

- 1 tablespoon olive oil
- 1 sweet onion, chopped, or about 1 cup precut packaged onion
- 1 teaspoon bottled minced garlic
- 1 teaspoon grated fresh ginger
- 2 cups finely chopped cauliflower
- 2 cups shredded broccoli stalks, or packaged broccoli slaw
- 1 cup shredded sweet potato
- 1 carrot, shredded, or ½ preshredded packaged carrots
- 1 cup peas (fresh or frozen and thawed)
- 1 cup chopped fresh spinach
- 2 tablespoons apple cider vinegar
- 1 teaspoon ground cumin
- ½ teaspoon ground coriander
- ¼ cup pumpkin seeds
- ¼ cup dried cherries
- 4 large cabbage leaves

1. Place a large skillet over medium-high heat and add the olive oil.
2. Add the onion, garlic, and ginger. Sauté for about 3 minutes, or until softened.
3. Stir in the cauliflower, broccoli, sweet potato, and carrot. Sauté for about 8 minutes, or until the vegetables are tender.
4. Stir in the peas, spinach, cider vinegar, cumin, and coriander. Sauté for about 2 minutes more until the spinach has wilted. Remove the skillet from the heat.
5. Stir in the pumpkin seeds and dried cherries. Spoon the vegetable mixture into the cabbage leaves and serve.

PER SERVING

Calories 208| Total fat 8g| Saturated fat 1g| Carbohydrates 29g| Fiber 8g| Protein 8g

Wild Mushroom Frittata

Prep time: 10 minutes|Cooking time:40 minutes|Serves 6-8

- 10 eggs
- ½ cup unsweetened almond milk
- ½ teaspoon ground cumin
- ½ teaspoon ground coriander
- ¼ teaspoon sea salt
- 1 tablespoon olive oil
- 2 cups sliced wild mushrooms
- ½ sweet onion, chopped, or about ½ cup precut packaged onion
- 2 teaspoons bottled minced garlic
- 1 tablespoon chopped fresh oregano

1. Preheat the oven to 350°F.
2. In a medium bowl, whisk the eggs, almond milk, cumin, coriander, and sea salt. Set it aside.
3. Place a large ovenproof skillet over medium-high heat and add the olive oil.
4. Add the mushrooms, onion, and garlic. Sauté for about 8 minutes, or until lightly caramelized.
5. Pour in the egg mixture and tap the skillet on the counter so the eggs flow into the vegetables.
6. Bake the frittata for about 30 minutes, or until it is cooked through and lightly browned.
7. Sprinkle with the oregano and serve.

PER SERVING

Calories 207| Total fat 15g| Saturated fat 4g| Carbohydrates 5g| Fiber 1g| Protein 15g

Pumpkin Curry

Prep time: 20 minutes|Cooking time:40 minutes|Serves 4

- 1 tablespoon olive oil
- 1 sweet onion, chopped, or about 1 cup precut packaged onion
- 2 teaspoons grated fresh ginger
- 6 cups (1-inch) pumpkin chunks
- 1 cup low-sodium vegetable broth
- 1 cup canned full-fat coconut milk
- 2 parsnips, diced, or 1 to 1½ cups precut packaged parsnips
- 1 carrot, diced, or ¾ cup precut packaged carrots
- 1 sweet potato, peeled and cut into 1-inch chunks, or 1½ cups precut packaged sweet potatoes
- 2 tablespoons Mild Curry Powder
- 2 cups quartered bok choy
- 2 tablespoons chopped fresh cilantro

1. Place a large saucepan over medium-high heat and add the olive oil.
2. Add the onion and ginger. Sauté for about 3 minutes, or until softened.
3. Stir in the pumpkin, vegetable broth, coconut milk, parsnips, carrot, sweet potato, and curry powder. Bring the liquid to a boil. Reduce the heat to low and simmer for about 30 minutes, stirring occasionally, until the vegetables are

tender and the sauce is thick and flavorful.
4. Stir in the bok choy and cook for about 5 minutes, stirring until it is tender.
5. Serve the curry topped with the cilantro.

PER SERVING

Calories 408| Total fat 20g| Saturated fat 14g| Carbohydrates 59g| Fiber 19g| Protein 8g

Simple Spaghetti Squash

Prep time: 15 minutes|Cooking time:8 hours|Serves 4 to 6

- 1 spaghetti squash, washed well
- 2 cups water

1. Using a fork, poke 10 to 15 holes all around the outside of the spaghetti squash.
2. Put the squash and the water in your slow cooker.
3. Cover the cooker and set to low. Cook for 8 hours.
4. Transfer the squash from the slow cooker to a cutting board.
5. Let sit for 15 minutes to cool.
6. Halve the squash lengthwise. Using a spoon, scrape the seeds out of the center of the squash.
7. Then, using a fork, scrape at the flesh until it shreds into a spaghetti-like texture.
8. Serve warm.

PER SERVING

Calories 60| Total Fat 0g| Total Carbs 15g| Sugar 0g| Fiber 0g| Protein 0g| Sodium 42mg

Stuffed Sweet Potatoes

Prep time: 15 minutes|Cooking time:6 to 7 hours|Serves 4

- 4 medium sweet potatoes
- 1 cup Hatch Chile "Refried" Beans
- 4 tablespoons chopped scallions (both white and green parts)
- 1 avocado, peeled, pitted, and quartered

1. Wash the sweet potatoes, but do not dry them.
2. The water left on the skins from washing is the only moisture needed for cooking.
3. Put the damp sweet potatoes in your slow cooker.
4. Cover the cooker and set to low.
5. Cook for 6 to 7 hours.
6. Carefully remove the hot sweet potatoes from the slow cooker.
7. Slice each one lengthwise about halfway through.
8. Mash the revealed flesh with a fork, and fill the opening with ¼ cup of beans.
9. Top each with 1 tablespoon of scallions and a quarter of the avocado and serve.

PER SERVING

Calories 237| Total Fat 8g| Total Carbs 38g| Sugar 7g| Fiber 10g| Protein 6g| Sodium 315mg

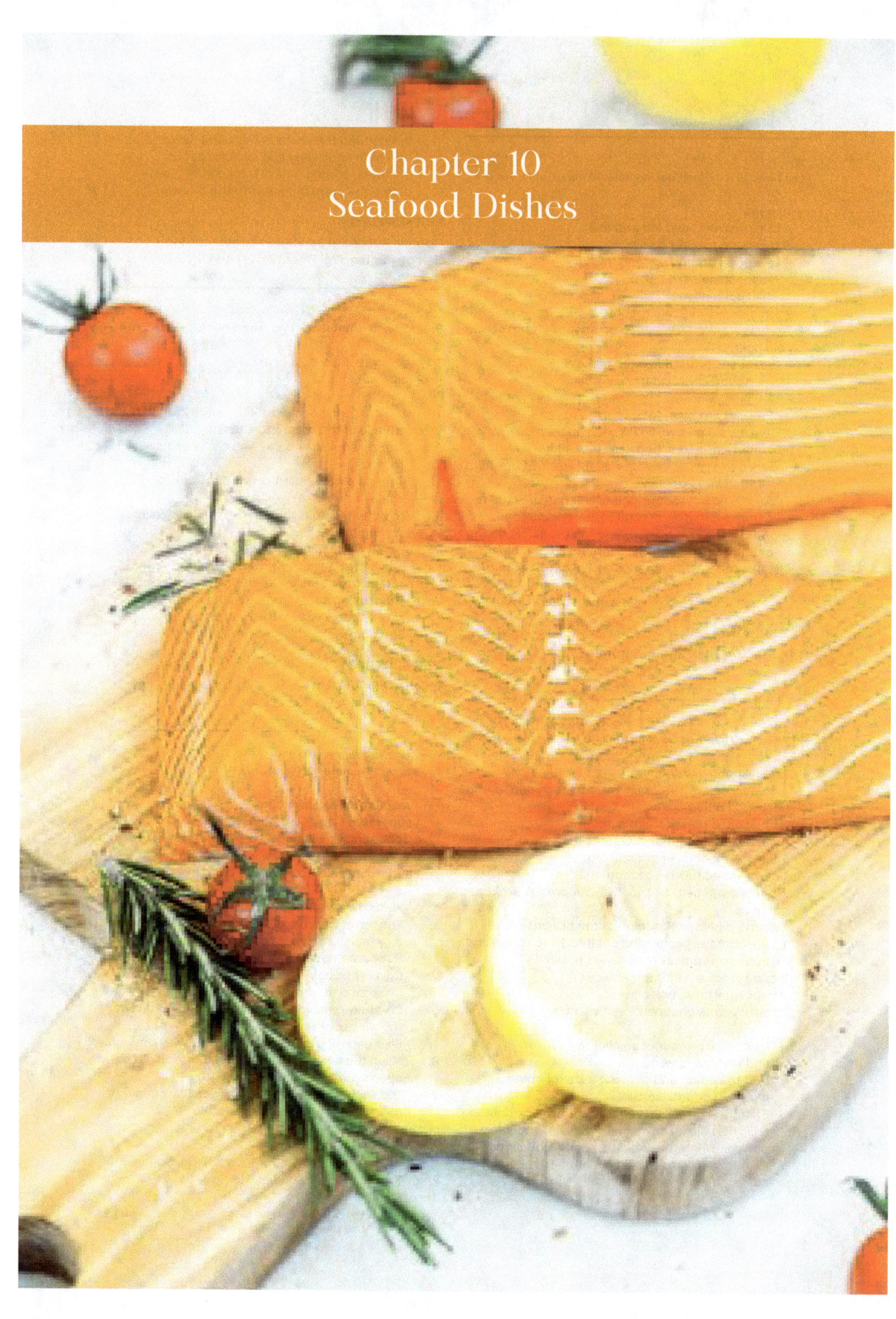

Chapter 10
Seafood Dishes

Tilapia Fish Tacos With Cilantro-Lime Crema

Prep time: 15 minutes|Cooking time:8 minutes|Serves 4

- For the cilantro-lime crema
- ½ cup plain whole-milk Greek yogurt
- 2 tablespoons freshly squeezed lime juice
- 1 tablespoon minced fresh cilantro leaves
- ¼ teaspoon garlic powder
- Dash salt
- For the fish tacos
- 8 small corn tortillas
- 1 teaspoon paprika
- ½ teaspoon salt
- ½ teaspoon garlic powder
- ½ teaspoon ground cumin
- ¼ teaspoon cayenne pepper
- 1 pound tilapia fillets
- 2 tablespoons avocado oil
- 1 large avocado, sliced

TO MAKE THE CILANTRO-LIME CREMA

1. In a small bowl, whisk the yogurt, lime juice, cilantro, garlic powder, and salt.
2. Cover and chill until ready to serve.

TO MAKE THE FISH TACOS

1. Preheat the oven to 350°F.
2. Wrap the tortillas in aluminum foil and place them in the oven to warm for about 15 minutes.
3. Meanwhile, in a small bowl, mix the paprika, salt, garlic powder, cumin, and cayenne pepper.
4. Put the fish fillets on a plate, and sprinkle them with the seasoning mixture.
5. In a large skillet over medium-high heat, heat the avocado oil.
6. Add the fish fillets to the skillet. Cook for 3 minutes per side, or until flaky.
7. Lay the warm tortillas out on a work surface. Divide the fish among the tortillas.
8. Serve the fish tacos with the sliced avocado and cilantro-lime crema.

PER SERVING

Calories 363| Total Fat 17g| Saturated Fat 3g| Cholesterol 62mg| Carbohydrates 25g| Fiber 6g| Protein 27g

Open-Face Avocado Tuna Melts

Prep time: 10 minutes|Cooking time:5 minutes|Serves 6-8

- 4 slices sourdough bread
- 2 (5-ounce) cans wild-caught albacore tuna
- ¼ cup Paleo mayonnaise
- 2 tablespoons minced shallot
- 1 teaspoon freshly squeezed lemon juice
- Dash garlic powder
- Dash paprika
- 1 large avocado, cut in 8 slices
- 1 large tomato, cut in 8 slices
- ¼ cup shredded raw Parmesan cheese, divided

1. Preheat the broiler.
2. Line a baking sheet with aluminum foil.
3. Arrange the slices of bread in the prepared pan.
4. In a medium bowl, mix the tuna, mayonnaise, shallot, lemon juice, garlic powder, and paprika. Spread one-fourth of the tuna mixture on each slice of bread.
5. Top each with 2 of the avocado slices and 2 of the tomato slices.
6. Sprinkle each with 1 tablespoon of Parmesan cheese.
7. Broil for 3 to 4 minutes, watching carefully so they don't burn. Serve hot.

PER SERVING

Calories 471| Total Fat 27g| Saturated Fat 4g| Cholesterol 40mg| Carbohydrates 31g| Fiber 4g| Protein 27g

Mediterranean Baked Salmon

Prep time: 5 minutes|Cooking time:20 minutes|Serves 4

- 4 (4-ounce) salmon fillets
- 3 tablespoons Pistachio Pesto
- ¼ cup chopped sun-dried tomatoes
- ¼ cup pitted, diced olives
- 2 tablespoons minced red onion
- 2 garlic cloves, minced
- Dash salt
- Fresh ground black pepper
- 1 tablespoon minced fresh basil

1. Preheat the oven to 400°F.
2. Line a baking sheet with aluminum foil.
3. Put the salmon fillets in the prepared pan, skin-side down.
4. Spread a thin layer of the pistachio pesto over the top of each fillet.
5. In a small bowl, mix the sun-dried tomatoes, olives, red onion, garlic, and salt, and season with pepper. Spread one-fourth of the tomato mixture over the pesto on each fillet.
6. Bake for 20 minutes. Remove from the oven and let rest for 5 minutes.
7. Sprinkle with the basil and serve immediately.

PER SERVING

Calories 301| Total Fat 17g| Saturated Fat 2g| Cholesterol 80mg| Carbohydrates 6g| Fiber 1g| Protein 31g

Saucy Oregon Bay Shrimp

Prep time: 20 minutes|Cooking time:10 minutes|Serves 4

- 2 tbsp olive oil
- 1 ½ lb Oregon Bay shrimp
- 2 tbsp Dijon mustard
- 1 cup chicken broth
- 2 tbsp parsley, chopped
- 1 tsp onion powder
- Sea salt and pepper to taste

1. Warm the olive oil in a skillet over medium heat and place in the shrimp. Stir-fry for 4 minutes until opaque.
2. Mix the mustard, chicken broth, parsley, onion powder, salt, and pepper in a bowl, pour it over the shrimp, and cook for another 3 minutes.
3. Serve immediately.

PER SERVING

Cal 280| Fat 12g| Carbs 5g| Protein 1g

Rosemary Salmon with Orange Glaze

Prep time: 10 minutes|Cooking time:30 minutes|Serves 4

- 2 tsp chopped rosemary
- 2 oranges, juiced
- 1 orange, zested
- ¼ cup pure maple syrup
- 2 tsp low-sodium soy sauce
- 1 tsp garlic powder
- 4 salmon fillets

1. Preheat your oven to 400°F.
2. Mix the orange juice, orange zest, maple syrup, soy sauce, and garlic powder in a bowl.
3. Add in salmon pieces, flesh-side down, and let marinate for 10 minutes. Transfer each piece skin-side up to a lined baking sheet and bake for 15 minutes until the salmon is lightly browned.
4. Garnish with rosemary and serve.

PER SERVING

Cal 300| Fat 12| Carbs 19g| Protein 1g

Roasted Salmon and Asparagus

Prep time: 5 minutes|Cooking time:15 minutes|Serves 4

- 1 pound asparagus spears, trimmed
- 2 tablespoons extra-virgin olive oil
- 1 teaspoon sea salt, divided
- 1½ pound salmon, cut into four fillets
- ⅛ teaspoon freshly cracked black pepper
- zest and slices from 1 lemon

1. Preheat the oven to 425°F.
2. Toss the asparagus with the olive oil and ½ teaspoon of the salt. Spread in a single layer in the bottom of a roasting pan.
3. Season the salmon with the pepper and remaining ½ teaspoon of salt. Place skin-side down on top of the asparagus.
4. Sprinkle the salmon and asparagus with the lemon zest and place the lemon slices over the fish.
5. Roast in the preheated oven 12 to 15 minutes, until the flesh is opaque.

PER SERVING

Calories 308| Total Fat 18g| Total Carbs 5g| Sugar 2g| Fiber 2g| Protein 36g| Sodium 545mg

Citrus Salmon on a Bed of Greens

Prep time: 10 minutes|Cooking time:19 minutes|Serves 4

- ¼ cup extra-virgin olive oil, divided
- 1½ pounds salmon
- 1 teaspoon sea salt, divided
- ½ teaspoon freshly ground black pepper, divided
- zest of 1 lemon
- 6 cups stemmed and chopped swiss chard
- 3 garlic cloves, minced
- juice of 2 lemons

1. In a large nonstick skillet over medium-high heat, heat 2 tablespoons of the olive oil until it shimmers.
2. Season the salmon with ½ teaspoon of the salt, ¼ teaspoon of the pepper, and the lemon zest.
3. Add the salmon to the skillet, skin-side up, and cook for about 7 minutes until the flesh is opaque.
4. Flip the salmon and cook for 3 to 4 minutes to crisp the skin.
5. Set aside on a plate, tented with aluminum foil.
6. Return the skillet to the heat, add the remaining 2 tablespoons of olive oil, and heat it until it shimmers.
7. Add the Swiss chard. Cook for about 7 minutes, stirring occasionally, until soft.
8. Add the garlic. Cook for 30 seconds, stirring constantly.
9. Sprinkle in the lemon juice, the remaining ½ teaspoon of salt, and the remaining ¼ teaspoon of pepper. Cook for 2 minutes.
10. Serve the salmon on the Swiss chard.

PER SERVING

Calories 363| Total Fat 25| Total Carbs 3g| Sugar <1g| Fiber 1g| Protein 34g| Sodium 662mg

Salmon Ceviche

Prep time: 10 minutes|Cooking time:20 minutes|Serves 4

- 1 pound salmon, skin and pin bones removed, cut into bite-size pieces (remove any gray flesh)
- ½ cup freshly squeezed lime juice
- 2 tomatoes, diced
- ¼ cup fresh cilantro leaves, chopped
- 1 jalapeño pepper, seeded and diced
- 2 tablespoons extra-virgin olive oil
- ½ teaspoon sea salt

1. In a medium bowl, stir together the salmon and lime juice. Let it marinate for 20 minutes.
2. Stir in the tomatoes, cilantro, jalapeño, olive oil, and salt.

PER SERVING

Calories 222| Total Fat 14g| Total Carbs 3g| Sugar 2g| Fiber <1g| Protein 23g| Sodium 288mg

Autenthic Salmon Ceviche

Prep time: 10 minutes|Cooking time:30 minutes|Serves 4

- 1 lb salmon, cubed
- 1 lime, juiced
- 1 Spanish onion, chopped
- 2 tomatoes, diced
- ¼ cup cilantro, chopped
- 1 jalapeño pepper, diced
- 2 tbsp olive oil
- ½ tsp sea salt

1. Mix the salmon and lemon juice and let marinate for 20 minutes.
2. Stir in onion, tomatoes, cilantro, jalapeño, olive oil, and salt.
3. Serve and enjoy!

PER SERVING

Cal 230| Fat 15g| Carbs 4g| Protein 1g

Mango Halibut Curry

Prep time: 10 minutes|Cooking time:20 minutes|Serves 4

- 1 tbsp olive oil
- 2 tbsp mango chutney
- 2 tsp ground turmeric
- 2 tsp curry powder
- 1 ½ lb halibut, cubed
- 4 cups chicken broth
- 1 (14-oz) can coconut milk
- Sea salt and pepper to taste
- 2 tbsp cilantro, chopped
- 1 red chili pepper, sliced

1. Warm the olive oil in a skillet over medium heat and place in the turmeric and curry powder and cook for 2 minutes.
2. Stir in halibut, chicken broth, coconut milk, mango chutney, salt, and pepper. Bring to a simmer, then cook for 6-7 minutes over low heat until the halibut is opaque and cooked through.
3. Spoon into bowls and top with finely chopped cilantro and chili slices.
4. Enjoy!

PER SERVING

Cal 430| Fat 48g| Carbs 6g| Protein 1g

Hawaiian Tuna

Prep time: 10 minutes|Cooking time:35 minutes|Serves 4

- 2 lb tuna, cubed
- 1 cup pineapple chunks
- ¼ cup chopped cilantro
- 2 tbsp chopped parsley
- 2 garlic cloves, minced
- 1 tbsp coconut oil
- 1 tbsp coconut aminos
- Sea salt and pepper to taste

1. Preheat your oven to 400°F.
2. Add the tuna, pineapple, cilantro, parsley, garlic, coconut aminos, salt, and pepper to a baking dish and stir to coat.
3. Bake for 15-20 minutes, or until the fish feels firm to the touch.
4. Serve warm.

PER SERVING

Cal 410| Fat 15g| Carbs 7g| Protein 59g

Almond-Crusted Tilapia

Prep time: 10 minutes|Cooking time:20 minutes|Serves 4

- 4 tilapia fillets
- 2 tbsp sliced almonds
- 2 tbsp Dijon mustard
- 1 tsp olive oil
- ¼ tsp black pepper

1. Pour 1 cup of water in your Instant Pot.
2. Mix the olive oil, pepper, and mustard in a small bowl.
3. Brush the fish fillets with the mustardy mixture on all sides.
4. Coat the fish in almonds slices.
5. Place the rack in your pot and arrange the fish fillets on it.
6. Close the lid and cook for 5 minutes on "Manual" setting on High pressure.
7. Do a quick pressure release and serve immediately.

PER SERVING

Cal 330| Fat 15g| Carbs 4g| Protein 46g

Asian-Inspired Salmon

Prep time: 10 minutes|Cooking time:15 minutes|Serves 4

- 3 tbsp miso paste
- 1 tsp coconut aminos
- 4 salmon fillets
- 2 tbsp honey
- 1 tsp rice vinegar

1. Preheat your broiler. Line a baking dish with foil. Place the salmon fillets on the baking dish.
2. In a bowl, combine miso paste, honey, coconut aminos, and rice vinegar.
3. Rub each fillet with this mixture and broil for 5 minutes.
4. Turn the fillets and rub with the remaining glaze and broil for 5 more minutes.
5. Serve immediately.

PER SERVING

Cal 265| Fat 11g| Carbs 15g| Protein 30g| Fiber 2g

Cod in Tomato Sauce

Prep time: 10 minutes|Cooking time:15 minutes|Serves 4

- 4 cod fillets
- 2 cups chopped tomatoes
- 1 tbsp olive oil
- Sea salt and pepper to taste
- ¼ tsp garlic powder

1. Place the tomatoes in a baking dish and crush them with a fork.
2. Season with some salt, pepper, and garlic powder.
3. Season the cod with salt and pepper and place it over the tomatoes.
4. Drizzle the olive oil over the fish and tomatoes.
5. Add 1 cup of water and a trivet in your Instant Pot.
6. Place the baking dish on the trivet.
7. Close the lid and cook on "Manual" for 10 minutes.
8. Once the timer goes off, let the steam release naturally for about 10 minutes before releasing the remaining pressure manually.
9. Serve.

PER SERVING

Cal 250| Fat 5g| Carbs 3g| Protein 45g

Curried Poached Halibut

Prep time: 5 minutes|Cooking time:23 minutes|Serves 4

- 1 tablespoon avocado oil
- ½ cup diced white onion
- 2 garlic cloves, minced
- 1 tablespoon red curry paste
- 1½ cups chicken broth
- 1 (14-ounce) can coconut milk
- ½ teaspoon coconut sugar
- 1 teaspoon salt
- ½ teaspoon freshly ground black pepper
- 4 (4-ounce) halibut fillets

1. In a large skillet over medium heat, heat the avocado oil.
2. Add the onion and garlic, and sauté for 2 to 3 minutes until the onions are translucent.
3. Stir in the curry paste until incorporated.
4. Add the broth, coconut milk, coconut sugar, salt, and pepper and stir to combine. Reduce the heat to medium-low and gently simmer for 10 minutes.
5. Pat the halibut dry with a paper towel. Place each fillet into the curried broth. Cover and poach for 10 minutes. Check the fish for doneness; if it flakes, it should be done. To speed the cooking time, occasionally spoon some broth over the halibut as it cooks.
6. Serve the fillets in four bowls with the curried broth spooned on top.

PER SERVING

Calories 358| Total Fat 22g| Saturated Fat 17g| Cholesterol 68mg| Carbohydrates 10g| Fiber 1g| Protein 28g

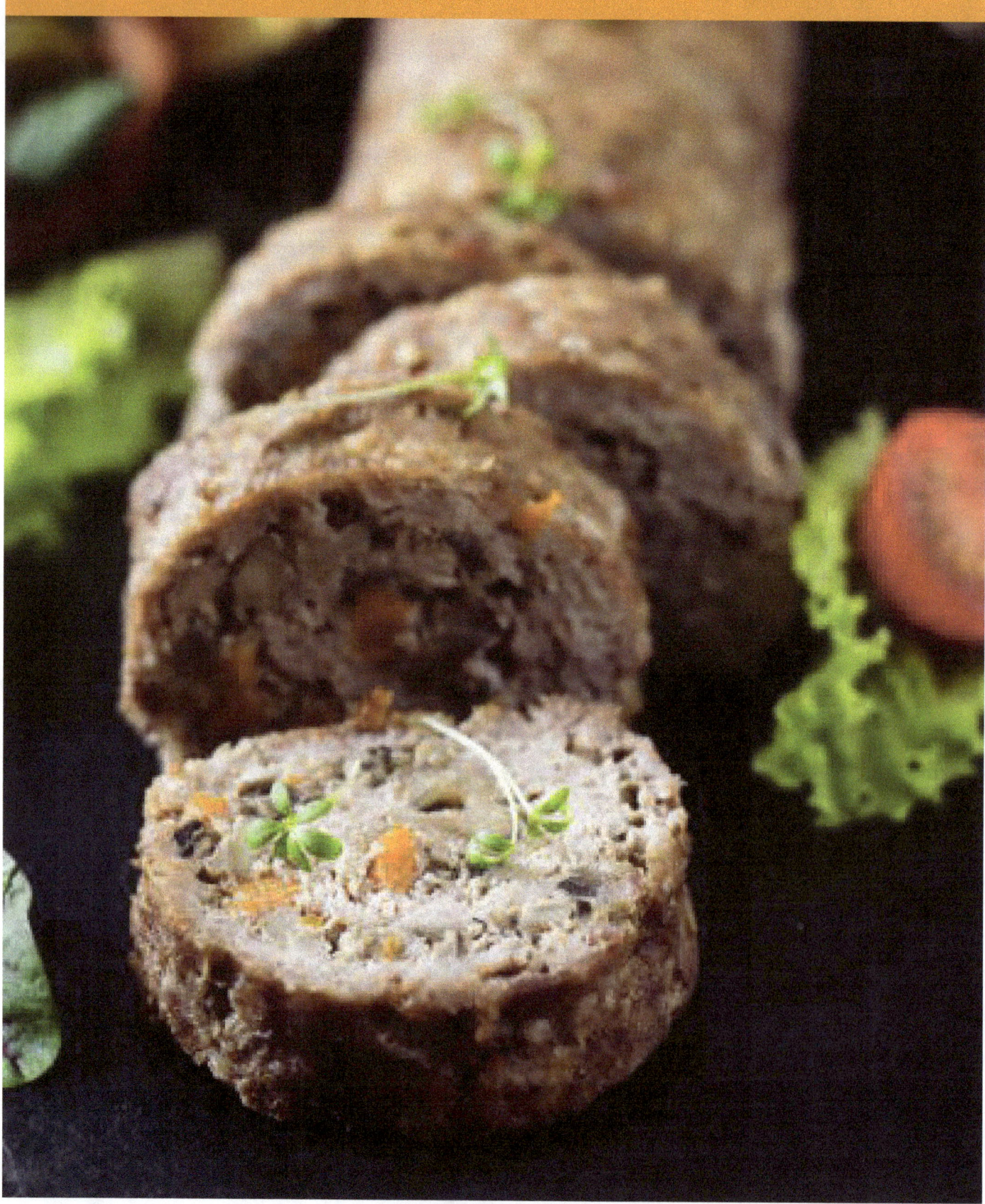

Turkey Larb Lettuce Wraps

Prep time: 10 minutes|Cooking time:20 minutes|Serves 4

- 1 pound ground turkey
- 1 small red onion, diced
- 2 garlic cloves, minced
- 4 scallions, sliced
- 2 tablespoons freshly squeezed lime juice
- 2 tablespoons fish sauce
- 2 tablespoons minced fresh cilantro
- 1 tablespoon minced fresh mint (optional)
- 1 tablespoon coconut sugar
- ¼ teaspoon red pepper flakes
- 8 small romaine lettuce leaves

1. In a large skillet over medium-high heat, cook the turkey for 10 minutes, stirring and breaking up the meat.
2. Add the onion and garlic, and cook for about 10 minutes, stirring, until the onions soften and the meat is cooked.
3. Remove from the heat. Stir in the scallions, lime juice, fish sauce, cilantro, mint (if using), coconut sugar, and red pepper flakes until well incorporated.
4. Fill each romaine leaf with the meat mixture.
5. Serve warm or cold.

PER SERVING

Calories 143| Total Fat 2g| Saturated Fat 1g| Cholesterol 70mg| Carbohydrates 9g| Fiber 1g| Protein 24g

Spicy Spinach-Turkey Burgers

Prep time: 10 minutes|Cooking time:12 minutes|Serves 4

- 2 cups fresh spinach, washed
- ⅓ small white onion, diced
- 1 egg, whisked
- 1 pound ground turkey
- 1 teaspoon garlic powder
- ½ teaspoon dried oregano
- ½ teaspoon dried basil
- ½ teaspoon red pepper flakes
- ½ teaspoon salt
- ¼ teaspoon dried thyme
- ¼ teaspoon freshly ground black pepper
- Dash cayenne pepper
- 1 tablespoon avocado oil

1. In a food processor (or blender), combine the spinach, onion, and egg. Pulse for about 15 seconds until the vegetables are minced.
2. Add the turkey, garlic powder, oregano, basil, red pepper flakes, salt, thyme, black pepper, and cayenne pepper. Pulse for 20 to 30 seconds until well combined.
3. Form the turkey mixture into 4 patties.
4. In a large skillet over medium heat, add the avocado oil. Cook the patties for about 6 minutes per side.

PER SERVING

Calories 197| Total Fat 11g| Saturated Fat 3g| Cholesterol 133mg| Carbohydrates 3g| Fiber 1g| Protein 23g

Turkey Meatballs In A Muffin Tin

Prep time: 10 minutes|Cooking time:20 minutes|Serves 12

- 1½ pounds ground turkey
- 1 small white onion, minced
- 1 egg, whisked
- ¼ cup fresh mushrooms, minced
- 1 teaspoon garlic powder
- ½ teaspoon salt
- ½ teaspoon dried oregano
- ¼ teaspoon freshly ground black pepper
- ¼ teaspoon ground ginger
- 1 slice gluten-free bread, torn into small pieces

1. Preheat the oven to 400°F.
2. In a large bowl, add the turkey, onion, egg, mushrooms, garlic powder, salt, oregano, pepper, ginger, and bread, and mix thoroughly with your hands.
3. Form the turkey mixture into 12 balls and place 1 in each cup of a 12-cup muffin tin.
4. Bake for 20 minutes.
5. Serve immediately.

PER SERVING

Calories 78| Total Fat 3g| Saturated Fat 0g| Cholesterol 26mg| Carbohydrates 3g| Fiber 0g| Protein 15g

Southwest Turkey-Stuffed Bell Peppers

Prep time: 10 minutes|Cooking time:20 minutes|Serves 6

- 6 bell peppers, any color, tops and ribs removed, seeded
- 1 tablespoon avocado oil
- 1 pound ground turkey
- 1 small white onion, diced
- 2 garlic cloves, minced
- 1 (16-ounce) can diced tomatoes, drained
- ½ teaspoon ground cumin
- ½ teaspoon paprika
- ½ teaspoon dried oregano
- ½ teaspoon salt
- Freshly ground black pepper

1. Preheat the oven to 400°F.
2. Line a baking sheet with aluminum foil.
3. Arrange the bell peppers on the prepared pan. Drizzle with the avocado oil.
4. Bake for 20 minutes, or until softened and cooked.
5. Meanwhile, in a large skillet over medium-high heat, brown the turkey for 5 minutes, breaking up the meat with a spoon.
6. Add the onion and garlic. Cook for 10 minutes, stirring frequently, until the turkey is cooked.
7. Stir in the tomatoes, cumin, paprika, oregano, and salt, and season with pepper.
8. Fill each cooked pepper with the meat mixture.
9. Enjoy warm.

PER SERVING

Calories 188| Total Fat 9g| Saturated Fat 2g| Cholesterol 60mg| Carbohydrates 11g| Fiber 4g| Protein 15g

Lamb & Quinoa Skillet Ragù

Prep time: 10 minutes|Cooking time:20 minutes|Serves 6

- 1 cup quinoa, rinsed well
- 2 cups filtered water
- 1 pound ground lamb
- 3 garlic cloves, minced
- 1 yellow onion, diced
- 1 red bell pepper, diced
- 1 (28-ounce) can diced tomatoes with their juice
- 1 cup minced fresh spinach leaves
- 2 teaspoons chili powder
- ½ teaspoon ground cumin
- ½ teaspoon smoked paprika
- Dash red pepper flakes

1. In a medium saucepan over high heat, bring the quinoa and the water to a boil.
2. Cover the pan and reduce the heat to low.
3. Simmer for 15 minutes. Remove from the heat and fluff with a fork.
4. Meanwhile, in a large skillet over medium heat, cook the lamb for 10 minutes, stirring occasionally to break up the meat.
5. Add the garlic, onion, and red bell pepper.
6. Cook, stirring, for 5 minutes.
7. Stir in the tomatoes, spinach, chili powder, cumin, paprika, and red pepper flakes.
8. Cover and cook for about 5 minutes, or until the lamb is fully cooked.
9. Remove the ragù from the heat and spoon over portions of quinoa.

PER SERVING

Calories 306| Total Fat 13g| Saturated Fat 5g| Cholesterol 50mg| Carbohydrates 26g| Fiber 5g| Protein 19g

Sweet Spiced Pecans

Prep time: 4 minutes|Cooking time:17 minutes|Serves 4

- 1 cup pecan halves
- ¼ cup packed brown sugar
- 3 tablespoons unsalted butter, melted
- 1 teaspoon ground cinnamon
- ½ teaspoon ground nutmeg
- ¼ teaspoon sea salt

1. Preheat the oven to 350°F.
2. Line a rimmed baking sheet with parchment paper.
3. In a medium bowl, toss together the pecans, brown sugar, butter, cinnamon, nutmeg, and salt to combine. Spread the nuts in a single layer on the prepared sheet.
4. Bake for 15 to 17 minutes until the nuts are fragrant.

PER SERVING

Calories 323| Total Fat 30g| Total Carbs 14g| Sugar 10g| Fiber 4g| Protein 3g| Sodium 181mg

Honeyed Apple Cinnamon Compote

Prep time: 15 minutes|Cooking time:10 minutes|Serves 4

- 6 apples, peeled, cored, and chopped
- ¼ cup apple juice
- ¼ cup honey
- 1 teaspoon ground cinnamon
- pinch sea salt

1. In a large pot over medium-high heat, combine the apples, apple juice, honey, cinnamon, and salt.
2. Simmer for about 10 minutes, stirring occasionally, until the apples are still quite chunky but also saucy.

PER SERVING

Calories 247| Total Fat <1g| Total Carbs 66g| Sugar 54g| Fiber 9g| Protein 1g| Sodium 63mg

Coconut Rice with Blueberries

Prep time: 15 minutes|Cooking time:10 minutes|Serves 4

- 1 (14-ounce) can full-fat coconut milk
- 1 cup fresh blueberries
- ¼ cup sugar
- 1 teaspoon ground ginger
- pinch sea salt
- 2 cups cooked brown rice

1. In a large pot over medium-high heat, combine the coconut milk, blueberries, sugar, ginger, and salt.
2. Cook for about 7 minutes, stirring constantly, until the blueberries soften.
3. Stir in the rice.
4. Cook for about 3 minutes, stirring, until the rice is heated through.

PER SERVING

Calories 469| Total Fat 25g| Total Carbs 60g| Sugar 19g| Fiber 5g| Protein 6g| Sodium 76mg

Herbed Lamb Fillets With Cauliflower Mash

Prep time: 10 minutes|Cooking time:15 minutes|Serves 4

- For the cauliflower mash
- 1 large head cauliflower, florets broken into small chunks
- Filtered water, for cooking the cauliflower
- 1 tablespoon ghee
- ½ teaspoon garlic powder
- ½ teaspoon salt
- Dash cayenne pepper
- For the lamb
- 2 (8-ounce) grass-fed lamb fillets
- 1 teaspoon salt
- ½ teaspoon freshly ground black pepper
- 2 tablespoons avocado oil
- 1 teaspoon dried rosemary

TO MAKE THE CAULIFLOWER MASH

1. In a large pot, combine the cauliflower and enough water to cover. Bring to a boil over high heat, and cook for 10 minutes.
2. Drain, and transfer to a food processor (or blender).
3. Add the ghee, garlic powder, salt, and cayenne pepper.
4. Pulse to a smooth consistency.

TO MAKE THE LAMB

1. Season the lamb with the salt and pepper.
2. In a large skillet over medium-high heat, add the avocado oil and rosemary.
3. Add the lamb fillets to the skillet, spaced so they are not touching. Sear for 5 minutes, spooning the rosemary oil from the bottom of the pan over the lamb halfway through. Flip and continue to cook the lamb for 5 minutes, basting with the rosemary oil after about 2 minutes.
4. Transfer to a plate, and let rest for 5 minutes.
5. Slice the lamb into coins and serve with the cauliflower mash.

PER SERVING

Calories 289| Total Fat 19g| Saturated Fat 7g| Cholesterol 74mg| Carbohydrates 8g| Fiber 3g| Protein 34g

Coconut-Curry-Cashew Chicken

Prep time: 15 minutes|Cooking time:7 to 8 hours|Serves 4 to 6

- 1½ cups Chicken Bone Broth
- 1 (14-ounce) can full-fat coconut milk
- 1 teaspoon garlic powder
- 1 tablespoon red curry paste
- 1 teaspoon sea salt
- ½ teaspoon freshly ground black pepper
- ½ teaspoon coconut sugar
- 2 pounds boneless, skinless chicken breasts
- 1½ cup unsalted cashews
- ½ cup diced white onion

1. In a medium bowl, combine the broth, coconut milk, garlic powder, red curry paste, salt, pepper, and coconut sugar. Stir well.
2. Put the chicken, cashews, and onion in the slow cooker.
3. Pour the coconut milk, mixture on top.
4. Cover the cooker and set to low.
5. Cook for 7 to 8 hours, or until the internal temperature of the chicken reaches 165°F on a meat thermometer and the juices run clear.
6. Shred the chicken with a fork, and mix it into the cooking liquid.
7. You can also remove the chicken from the broth and chop it with a knife into bite-size pieces before returning it to the slow cooker.
8. Serve.

PER SERVING

Calories 714| Total Fat 43g| Total Carbs 21g| Sugar 5g| Fiber 3g| Protein 57g| Sodium 1,606mg

Turkey & Sweet Potato Chili

Prep time: 15 minutes|Cooking time: 4 to 6 hours|Serves 4 to 6

- 1 tablespoon extra-virgin olive oil
- 1 pound ground turkey
- 3 cups sweet potato cubes
- 1 (28-ounce) can diced tomatoes
- 1 red bell pepper, diced
- 1 (4-ounce) can Hatch green chiles
- ½ medium red onion, diced
- 2 cups broth of choice
- 1 tablespoon freshly squeezed lime juice
- 1 tablespoon chili powder
- 1 teaspoon garlic powder
- 1 teaspoon cocoa powder
- 1 teaspoon ground cumin
- 1 teaspoon sea salt
- ½ teaspoon ground cinnamon
- Pinch cayenne pepper

1. In your slow cooker, combine the olive oil, turkey, sweet potato cubes, tomatoes, bell pepper, chiles, onion, broth, lime juice, chili powder, garlic powder, cocoa powder, cumin, salt, cinnamon, and cayenne.
2. Using a large spoon, break up the turkey into smaller chunks as it combines with the other ingredients.
3. Cover the cooker and set to low.
4. Cook for 4 to 6 hours.
5. Stir the chili well, continuing to break up the rest of the turkey, and serve.

PER SERVING

Calories 380| Total Fat 12g| Total Carbs 38g| Sugar 12g| Fiber 6g| Protein 30g| Sodium 1,268mg

Moroccan Turkey Tagine

Prep time: 15 minutes|Cooking time:7 to 8 hours|Serves 4 to 6

- 4 cups boneless, skinless turkey breast chunks
- 1 (14-ounce) can diced tomatoes
- 1 (14-ounce) can chickpeas, rinsed and drained well
- 2 large carrots, finely chopped
- ½ cup dried apricots
- ½ red onion, chopped
- 2 tablespoons raw honey
- 1 tablespoon tomato paste
- 1 teaspoon garlic powder
- 1 teaspoon ground turmeric
- ½ teaspoon sea salt
- ¼ teaspoon ground ginger
- ¼ teaspoon ground coriander
- ¼ teaspoon paprika
- ½ cup water
- 2 cups broth of choice
- Freshly ground black pepper

1. In your slow cooker, combine the turkey, tomatoes, chickpeas, carrots, apricots, onion, honey, tomato paste, garlic powder, turmeric, salt, ginger, coriander, paprika, water, and broth, and season with pepper.
2. Gently stir to blend the ingredients.
3. Cover the cooker and set to low.
4. Cook for 7 to 8 hours and serve.

PER SERVING

Calories 428| Total Fat 5g| Total Carbs 46g| Sugar 25g| Fiber 8g| Protein 49g| Sodium 983mg

Pork Tenderloin With Dijon-Cider Glaze

Prep time: 5 minutes|Cooking time:25 minutes|Serves 4

- ¼ cup apple cider vinegar
- ¼ cup coconut sugar
- 3 tablespoons Dijon mustard
- 2 teaspoons garlic powder
- Dash salt
- 1 (1½-pound) pork tenderloin

1. In a small bowl, stir together the vinegar, coconut sugar, mustard, garlic powder, and salt until the sugar dissolves.
2. Brush this mixture over the pork loin.
3. Place a grill pan over medium-high heat and add the pork.
4. Sear for 2 minutes per side.
5. Spoon half of the vinegar mixture over the pork and reduce the heat to medium.
6. Cover the pan and cook for 10 minutes.
7. Spoon the remaining vinegar mixture over the pork.
8. Cook for 5 minutes, or until the center of the pork reaches 145°F. Transfer the pork to a plate.
9. Bring the vinegar mixture remaining in the pan to a simmer.
10. Cook for 5 minutes to reduce and thicken.
11. Serve the pork drizzled with the glaze.

PER SERVING

Calories 268| Total Fat 6g| Saturated Fat 2g| Cholesterol 110mg| Carbohydrates 16g| Fiber 0g| Protein 36g

Thai Ground Beef With Asparagus & Chiles

Prep time: 10 minutes|Cooking time:17 minutes|Serves 4

- 1 tablespoon plus 1 teaspoon fish sauce
- 1 tablespoon plus 1 teaspoon coconut aminos
- 1 teaspoon coconut sugar
- 1 tablespoon coconut oil
- 1 bunch asparagus, tough ends trimmed, shaved into ribbons with a vegetable peeler
- 3 garlic cloves, minced
- 3 red jalapeño chile peppers, seeded and sliced into 2-inch matchsticks
- 1¼ pounds lean ground beef
- 1 cup loosely packed fresh basil leaves
- Lime wedges, for garnish

1. In a small bowl, stir together the fish sauce, coconut aminos, and coconut sugar. Set aside.
2. In a large skillet over medium heat, heat the coconut oil. Add the asparagus, and sauté for 1 minute. Transfer to a plate and set aside.
3. To the skillet, add the garlic and half of the jalapeño chiles. Cook for 15 seconds, stirring constantly.
4. Add the ground beef, and cook for about 15 minutes until cooked through and browned, breaking the meat up with a wooden spoon.
5. Stir in the sauce. Cook for 30 seconds.
6. Add the basil, cooked asparagus, and remaining half of the jalapeño chiles, and stir to combine.
7. Serve hot, garnished with lime wedges.

PER SERVING

Calories 214| Total Fat 13g| Saturated Fat 6g| Cholesterol 59mg| Carbohydrates 5g| Fiber 2g| Protein 21g

Spaghetti Bolognese

Prep time: 10 minutes|Cooking time:20 minutes|Serves 8

- 1 pound brown rice spaghetti
- 2 tablespoons ghee
- 3 garlic cloves, minced
- ½ cup chopped white onion
- ⅔ cup chopped celery
- ⅔ cup chopped carrot
- 1 pound lean ground beef
- 1 (14-ounce) can diced tomatoes with their juice
- 1 tablespoon white wine vinegar
- ½ teaspoon red pepper flakes
- ⅛ teaspoon ground nutmeg
- Dash salt
- Dash freshly ground black pepper

1. Cook the spaghetti according to the package instructions.
2. Meanwhile, in a large skillet over medium heat, heat the ghee.
3. Add the garlic and onion, and sauté for 5 minutes.
4. Add the celery and carrot, and sauté for 5 minutes. Push the vegetables to the side of the skillet.
5. Add the ground beef next to the vegetables. Sauté for 10 minutes, breaking up the meat as it begins to brown.
6. Stir in the tomatoes, vinegar, red pepper flakes, nutmeg, salt, and pepper, and bring to a simmer for 5 minutes.
7. Serve over the cooked noodles.

PER SERVING

Calories 358| Total Fat 12g| Saturated Fat 5g| Cholesterol 33mg| Carbohydrates 48g| Fiber 3g| Protein 14g

Sesame-Ginger Bok Choy & Beef Stir-Fry

Prep time: 10 minutes|Cooking time:10 minutes|Serves 4

- 12 ounces flank steak, cut into thin 2-inch strips
- ½ teaspoon salt
- ¼ teaspoon freshly ground black pepper
- 2 teaspoons avocado oil
- 1 tablespoon sesame oil
- 2 garlic cloves, minced
- 4 heads baby bok choy, quartered lengthwise
- 3 tablespoons coconut aminos
- 2 tablespoons rice vinegar
- 1 tablespoon grated peeled fresh ginger
- 1 tablespoon coconut sugar
- ¼ teaspoon red pepper flakes (optional)

1. Place a large skillet over medium-high heat.
2. Season the steak strips with the salt and pepper.
3. Add it to the skillet with the avocado oil, and stir-fry for 3 to 4 minutes until just cooked.
4. Transfer to a plate.
5. Wipe out the skillet.
6. Reduce the heat to medium and add the sesame oil and garlic.
7. Cook, stirring occasionally, for 2 to 3 minutes.
8. Stir in the bok choy, coconut aminos, vinegar, ginger, coconut sugar, and red pepper flakes (if using) until well combined.
9. Cover and cook for 2 minutes.
10. Add the steak to the skillet.
11. Toss gently to combine and warm through, about 1 minute.
12. Serve hot.

PER SERVING

Calories 252| Total Fat 13g| Saturated Fat 4g| Cholesterol 56mg| Carbohydrates 12g| Fiber 9g| Protein 19g

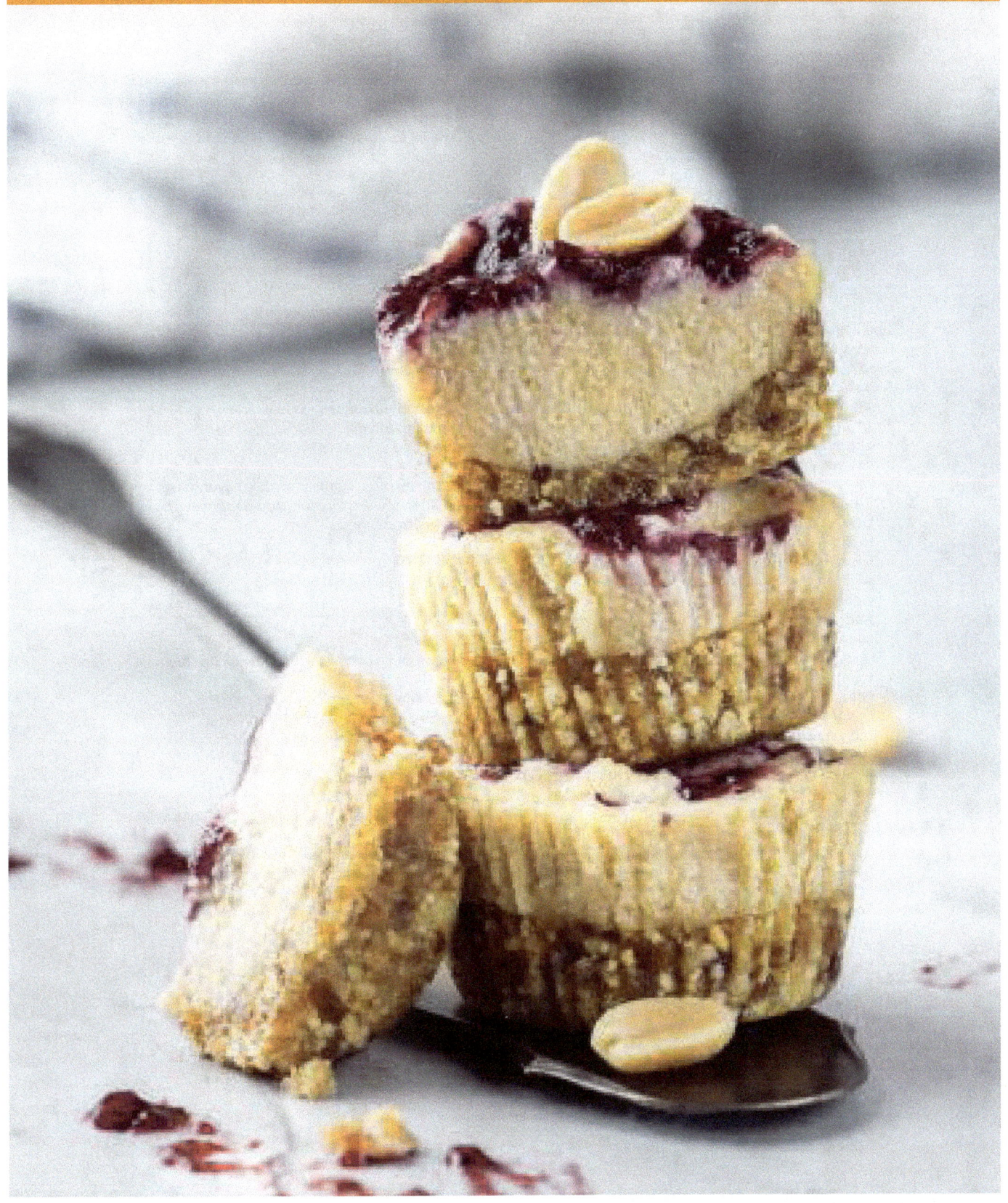

Banana "Nice" Cream

Prep time: 5 minutes|Cooking time:10 minutes|Serves 8

- 4 frozen, diced bananas

1. In a food processor or blender, blend the bananas for 3 to 5 minutes until they reach a whipped, creamy consistency.
2. Depending on how frozen the bananas are, it may take a bit longer.
3. Serve immediately.

PER SERVING

Calories 112| Total Fat 0g| Saturated Fat 0g| Cholesterol 0mg| Carbohydrates 29g| Fiber 3g| Protein 1g

Chewy Chocolate Chip Cookies

Prep time: 10 minutes|Cooking time:8 to 10 minutes|Serves 8

- 2 large eggs
- ⅓ cup granulated erythritol or other low-carb sweetener
- 1 teaspoon pure vanilla extract
- ⅓ cup plus 1 tablespoon coconut flour
- 1 tablespoon unflavored grass-fed beef gelatin
- ½ teaspoon baking soda
- Pinch of fine Himalayan salt
- 1 (4-ounce) bar stevia-sweetened semisweet baking chocolate, finely chopped, or ½ cup stevia-sweetened semisweet chocolate chips

1. Preheat the oven to 350°F.
2. Line a baking sheet with parchment paper.
3. In a large bowl, whisk the eggs with a fork or wire whisk until frothy.
4. Add the erythritol, butter, and vanilla extract and whisk until well combined.
5. Add the coconut flour, gelatin, baking soda, and salt to the wet ingredients.
6. Using a rubber spatula, mix the ingredients together until a dough forms.
7. Fold the chopped chocolate into the dough.
8. Using a medium-sized cookie scoop or a tablespoon, scoop up a mounded tablespoon of the dough and shape it into a 1-inch ball.
9. Repeat with the rest of dough, spacing the dough balls 2 inches apart on the lined baking sheet. (You should have a total of twelve.)
10. Using the palm of your hand, gently flatten the balls so they are about ½ inch thick.
11. Bake the cookies for 8 to 10 minutes, until the edges are lightly browned.
12. Remove the cookies from the oven and let cool to room temperature on the baking sheet before handling.
13. The more they cool, the chewier they will be.
14. Store in an airtight container at room temperature for up to 5 days.

PER SERVING

Calories 63 | Fat 4 3g | Total Carbohydrate 9 9g | Dietary Fiber 4 3g | Protein 2 9g

Garlicky Sweet Potatoes

Prep time: 10 minutes|Cooking time:25 minutes|Serves 4

- 2 tbsp extra-virgin olive oil
- 2 sweet potatoes, cubed
- 1 tbsp chopped oregano
- Sea salt and pepper to taste
- 3 garlic cloves, minced

1. Warm the olive oil in a skillet over medium heat and cook the sweet potatoes, oregano, and salt for 10-15 minutes until the potatoes get brown.
2. Add in garlic and pepper and cook for another 30 seconds.
3. Serve immediately.

PER SERVING

Cal 200| Fat 8g| Carbs 34g| Protein 2

Easy Homemade Ranch Dip

Prep time: 10 minutes|Cooking time:10 minutes|Serves 4

- ¼ cup sour cream
- ¼ cup mayonnaise
- ¼ garlic powder
- 1 tbsp chopped chives
- 1 tbsp chopped dill
- Sea salt and pepper to taste

1. Combine the sour cream, mayonnaise, garlic powder, chives, dill, salt, and pepper in a bowl until well combined.

PER SERVING

Cal 70| Fat 6g| Carbs 7g| Protein 1g

Chinese Cranberry Nut Trail Mix

Prep time: 10 minutes|Cooking time:10 minutes|Serves 4

- ½ tsp Chinese five-spice powder
- ½ cup dried cranberries
- 1 tbsp extra-virgin olive oil
- 1 cup almonds
- A pinch of sea salt

1. Warm the olive oil in a skillet over medium heat and cook the almonds, salt, and Chinese five-spice for 2 minutes, stirring often.
2. Turn the heat off and let cool before mixing in the ½ cup dried cranberries.
3. Serve.

PER SERVING

Cal 180| Fat 17g| Carbs 9g| Protein 4g

Spicy Mixed Nuts

Prep time: 10 minutes|Cooking time:10 minutes|Serves 6-8

- 1 cup almonds
- ½ cup walnuts
- 1 tsp ground turmeric
- ¼ cup sunflower seeds
- ¼ cup pumpkin puree
- ¼ tsp garlic powder
- ½ tsp ground cumin
- ¼ tsp red pepper flakes

1. Preheat the oven to 350°F.
2. Mix the 1 cup almonds, walnuts, turmeric, sunflower seeds, pumpkin puree, garlic powder, cumin, and red pepper flakes in a bowl.
3. Place the mixture on a baking sheet and bake for 15 minutes.
4. Let cool and store them.

PER SERVING

Cal 182| Fat 15g| Carbs 8g| Protein 6g| Fiber 5g

Butternut Squash Fries

Prep time: 20 minutes|Cooking time:40 to 45 minutes|-Serves 6-8

- 1 large butternut squash, peeled, seeded, and cut into fry-size pieces, about 3 inches long and ½ inch thick
- 2 tablespoons coconut oil
- ¾ teaspoon salt
- 3 fresh rosemary sprigs, stemmed and chopped (about 1½ tablespoons)

1. Preheat the oven to 375°F.
2. Line a large baking sheet with parchment paper or aluminum foil.
3. In a large bowl, toss the squash pieces with the coconut oil and salt. Scatter the butternut squash over the prepared sheet.
4. Place the sheet in the preheated oven and bake for 20 minutes. Flip the fries over.
5. Continue baking for 10 minutes more.
6. Sprinkle the fries with the rosemary. Bake for 10 to 15 minutes more, or until the fries are golden on the outside.
7. Serve hot.

PER SERVING

Calories 192| Total Fat 7g| Total Carbohydrates 34g| Sugar 6g| Fiber 7g| Protein 3g| Sodium 450mg

Homemade Trail Mix

Prep time: 5 minutes|Cooking time:0 minutes|Serves 12 to 14

- 1 cup pumpkin seeds
- 1 cup sunflower seeds
- 1 cup large coconut flakes
- 1 cup raisins
- 1 cup dried cranberries
- ½ cup cacao nibs (optional)

1. In a large bowl, stir together the pumpkin seeds, sunflower seeds, coconut, raisins, cranberries, and cacao nibs (if using).
2. Store, covered, in large jars in a cool, dry place, or portion into small containers for a quick grab-and-go option.

PER SERVING

Calories 183| Total Fat 11g| Total Carbohydrates 19g| Sugar 12g| Fiber 3g| Protein 5g| Sodium 24mg

Roasted Apricots

Prep time: 10 minutes|Cooking time:25 to 30 minutes minutes|Serves 8

- 20 fresh apricots, pitted and quartered
- 2 tablespoons coconut oil
- ⅛ teaspoon cardamom (optional)

1. Preheat the oven to 350°F.
2. In an ovenproof dish, toss the apricots with the coconut oil and cardamom (if using).
3. Place the dish in the preheated oven and roast for 25 to 30 minutes, stirring occasionally.

PER SERVING

Calories 142| Total Fat 8g| Total Carbohydrates 19g| Sugar 16g| Fiber 3g| Protein 2g| Sodium 2mg

Hot Cashew Hummus

Prep time: 10 minutes|Cooking time:20 minutes|Serves 6-8

- ¼ tsp sea salt
- 1 cup raw cashews
- 2 garlic cloves
- 1 tbsp extra-virgin olive oil
- 1 tsp lemon juice
- 2 tsp coconut aminos
- ½ tsp ground ginger
- ¼ tsp cayenne pepper

1. Soak the cashews in water for 15 minutes; drain.
2. Place the cashews, garlic, ¼ cup of water, olive oil, lemon juice, coconut aminos, ginger, cayenne pepper, and salt in a food processor and pulse until smooth.
3. Let chill in the fridge before serving.

PER SERVING

Cal 115| Fat 9g| Carbs 5g| Protein 3g| Fiber 2g

Mixed Bean Dip

Prep time: 5 minutes|Cooking time:10 minutes|Serves 10

- 14 oz canned kidney beans
- 4 oz canned black beans
- 2 Cherry tomatoes
- 2 garlic cloves
- 1 tbsp apple cider vinegar
- 2 tsp honey
- 1 tsp lime juice
- Sea salt and pepper to taste
- ¼ tsp ground cumin
- ¼ tsp cayenne pepper

1. Place the kidney beans, black beans, cherry tomatoes, garlic, 2 tbsp of water, apple cider vinegar, honey, lime juice, salt, cumin, cayenne pepper, and black pepper in a food processor and pulse until smooth.
2. Let chill.

PER SERVING

Cal 165| Fat 0,5g| Carbs 34g |Protein 9g| Fiber 3g

Coconut-Mango Lassi

Prep time: 10 minutes|Cooking time:10 minutes|Serves 6-8

- 1½ cups frozen mango chunks
- 1 cup unsweetened coconut milk
- 1 cup ice cubes
- ½ cup plain yogurt
- 1 tablespoon honey
- Pinch ground cardamom

1. Combine the mango, coconut milk, ice cubes, yogurt, and honey in a blender and blend until smooth.
2. Pour into two tall glasses. Sprinkle a little ground cardamom over each drink and serve.

PER SERVING

Calories 370| Total Fat 26g| Total Carbohydrates 32g| Sugar 27g| Fiber 2g| Protein 8g| Sodium 30mg

Avocado Fudge

Prep time: 15 minutes|Cooking time:10 minutes|Serves 16

- 1½ cup bittersweet chocolate chips
- ¼ cup coconut oil
- 1 ripe avocado, peeled and pitted
- ½ teaspoon sea salt

1. Line an 8-inch square baking pan with waxed or parchment paper.
2. In a double boiler (not the microwave), melt the chocolate and coconut oil.
3. Once melted, transfer to the bowl of a food processor and let them cool a bit. (If the chocolate is too hot when combined with the avocado, the mixture will separate.) Add the avocado and process until smooth.
4. Spoon the mixture into the lined pan, sprinkle with the sea salt, and chill for 3 hours. Cut into 16 pieces and serve.

PER SERVING

Calories 120| Total Fat 9g| Total Carbohydrates 11g| Sugar 9g| Fiber 2g| Protein 1g| Sodium 80mg

Coconut Citrus Tart

Prep time: 10 minutes|Cooking time:15 minutes|Serves 16

- 2 tablespoons ghee, unsalted butter, or lard
- 2 tablespoons granulated erythritol or other low-carb sweetener
- 1 (13.5-ounce) can full-fat coconut milk
- 1 teaspoon pure vanilla extract
- Grated zest of 1 lime or lemon, plus more for garnish
- Pinch of fine Himalayan salt
- 1 tablespoon unflavored grass-fed beef gelatin
- 1 Pie Crust, baked in an 8-inch springform pan
- 2 tablespoons unsweetened shredded coconut, for garnish

1. In a small saucepan over medium heat, melt the ghee.
2. Add the erythritol and let it simmer, stirring occasionally, until it melts into a syrup, about 10 minutes.
3. While the ghee mixture simmers, in a small bowl, whisk together the coconut milk, vanilla extract, citrus zest, and salt.
4. Quickly stir the coconut milk mixture into the syrup.
5. Cook for 5 to 8 minutes, until the mixture is steaming, almost at a simmer.
6. As you whisk vigorously, sprinkle in the gelatin. Stir until it's fully dissolved.
7. Slowly pour the coconut milk mixture into the prepared crust.
8. Place the tart on a plate or tray in case anything seeps from the springform pan.
9. Chill in the fridge for 4 hours, or until the center is completely set.
10. Garnish with more grated citrus zest and shredded coconut and serve. Wrap the leftovers in plastic wrap and store in the fridge for up to 3 days.

PER SERVING

Calories 142 | Fat 13.5g | Total Carbohydrate 4.4g | Dietary Fiber 1.4g | Protein 2.4g

Cortado Panna Cotta

Prep time: 5 minutes|Cooking time:10 minutes|Serves 4

- Espresso-grind dark-roast coffee
- ½ cup full-fat coconut milk
- 1 tablespoon granulated erythritol or other low-carb sweetener
- 1 tablespoon unflavored grass-fed beef gelatin
- Coconut Yogurt, for serving (optional)
- Special equipment:
- Moka pot or French press

1. Prepare your stovetop espresso using a moka pot or French press: Fill the bottom chamber with water up to the bolt or knob.
2. Fill the basket with the ground coffee, full but not too packed.
3. Place that over the chamber, then screw on the top.
4. Place the moka pot on a burner over medium-high heat.
5. The espresso will take a few minutes to brew, but keep your ears listening for the sound of rising water, when the pressure begins to build.
6. Heat the coconut milk in a small saucepan over medium heat.
7. Have the erythritol ready in a 2-cup glass measuring cup next to the stove, along with a teaspoon measuring spoon.
8. When the first drops of coffee come through the spout of the moka pot, measure 4 teaspoons into the measuring cup containing the sweetener.
9. Place the moka pot back on the stove to finish brewing.
10. Vigorously mix the sweetener and coffee into a sugary paste or syrup.
11. Once the coffee has finished brewing, the moka pot will be full; continue to beat the syrup as you pour the remaining coffee from the moka pot into the measuring cup.
12. Stir until fully combined.
13. Add the steamed coconut milk and then sprinkle in the gelatin as you continue to whisk the coffee mixture.
14. Set four 6-ounce glasses on a small tray and divide the coffee mixture equally among them.
15. Place in the fridge to cool and firm up for at least 2 hours.
16. Serve chilled with a dollop of coconut yogurt on top, if desired.

PER SERVING

Calories 75 | Fat 7.2g | Total Carbohydrate 1.7g | Dietary Fiber 0.7g | Protein 2.3g

Appendix 1 Measurement Conversion Chart

Volume Equivalents (Dry)

US STANDARD	METRIC (APPROXIMATE)
1/8 teaspoon	0.5 mL
1/4 teaspoon	1 mL
1/2 teaspoon	2 mL
3/4 teaspoon	4 mL
1 teaspoon	5 mL
1 tablespoon	15 mL
1/4 cup	59 mL
1/2 cup	118 mL
3/4 cup	177 mL
1 cup	235 mL
2 cups	475 mL
3 cups	700 mL
4 cups	1 L

Volume Equivalents (Liquid)

US STANDARD	US STANDARD (OUNCES)	METRIC (APPROXIMATE)
2 tablespoons	1 fl.oz.	30 mL
1/4 cup	2 fl.oz.	60 mL
1/2 cup	4 fl.oz.	120 mL
1 cup	8 fl.oz.	240 mL
1 1/2 cup	12 fl.oz.	355 mL
2 cups or 1 pint	16 fl.oz.	475 mL
4 cups or 1 quart	32 fl.oz.	1 L
1 gallon	128 fl.oz.	4 L

Temperatures Equivalents

FAHRENHEIT(F)	CELSIUS(C) APPROXIMATE
225 °F	107 °C
250 °F	120 ° °C
275 °F	135 °C
300 °F	150 °C
325 °F	160 °C
350 °F	180 °C
375 °F	190 °C
400 °F	205 °C
425 °F	220 °C
450 °F	235 °C
475 °F	245 °C
500 °F	260 °C

Weight Equivalents

US STANDARD	METRIC (APPROXIMATE)
1 ounce	28 g
2 ounces	57 g
5 ounces	142 g
10 ounces	284 g
15 ounces	425 g
16 ounces (1 pound)	455 g
1.5 pounds	680 g
2 pounds	907 g

Appendix 2 The Dirty Dozen and Clean Fifteen

The Environmental Working Group (EWG) is a nonprofit, nonpartisan organization dedicated to protecting human health and the environment Its mission is to empower people to live healthier lives in a healthier environment. This organization publishes an annual list of the twelve kinds of produce, in sequence, that have the highest amount of pesticide residue-the Dirty Dozen-as well as a list of the fifteen kinds of produce that have the least amount of pesticide residue-the Clean Fifteen.

THE DIRTY DOZEN	
The 2016 Dirty Dozen includes the following produce. These are considered among the year's most important produce to buy organic:	
Strawberries	Spinach
Apples	Tomatoes
Nectarines	Bell peppers
Peaches	Cherry tomatoes
Celery	Cucumbers
Grapes	Kale/collard greens
Cherries	Hot peppers
The Dirty Dozen list contains two additional itemskale/ collard greens and hot peppers-because they tend to contain trace levels of highly hazardous pesticides.	

THE CLEAN FIFTEEN	
The least critical to buy organically are the Clean Fifteen list. The following are on the 2016 list:	
Avocados	Papayas
Corn	Kiw
Pineapples	Eggplant
Cabbage	Honeydew
Sweet peas	Grapefruit
Onions	Cantaloupe
Asparagus	Cauliflower
Mangos	
Some of the sweet corn sold in the United States are made from genetically engineered (GE) seedstock. Buy organic varieties of these crops to avoid GE produce.	

Appendix 3 Index

MARILYN K. HAMILTON

Printed in the USA
CPSIA information can be obtained
at www.ICGtesting.com
LVHW070741111223
766178LV00018B/787